THE
MAGIC
OF INCLUSION

Give People A Chance
And Watch Them Shine

JULIE FISHER

First published by Ultimate World Publishing 2021
Copyright © 2021 Juile Fisher

ISBN

Paperback: 978-1-922597-53-3
Ebook: 978-1-922597-54-0

Juile Fisher has asserted her rights under the Copyright, Designs and Patents Act 1988 to be identified as the author of this work. The information in this book is based on the author's experiences and opinions. The publisher specifically disclaims responsibility for any adverse consequences which may result from use of the information contained herein. Permission to use information has been sought by the author. Any breaches will be rectified in further editions of the book.

All rights reserved. No part of this publication may be reproduced, stored in or introduced into a retrieval system, or transmitted in any form, or by any means (electronic, mechanical, photocopying, recording or otherwise) without the prior written permission of the author. Any person who does any unauthorised act in relation to this publication may be liable to criminal prosecution and civil claims for damages. Enquiries should be made through the publisher.

Cover design: Ultimate World Publishing
Layout and typesetting: Ultimate World Publishing
Editor: Marinda Wilkinson
Photographer: Tiny and Brave

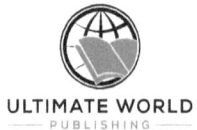

Ultimate World Publishing
Diamond Creek,
Victoria Australia 3089
www.writeabook.com.au

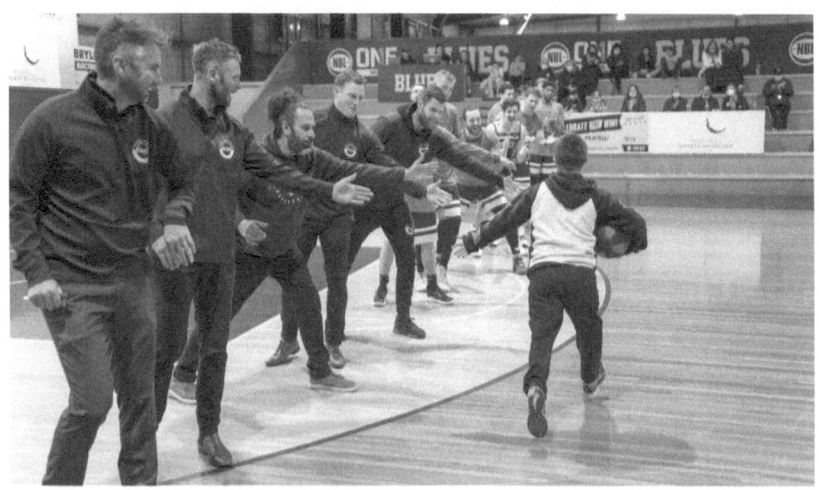

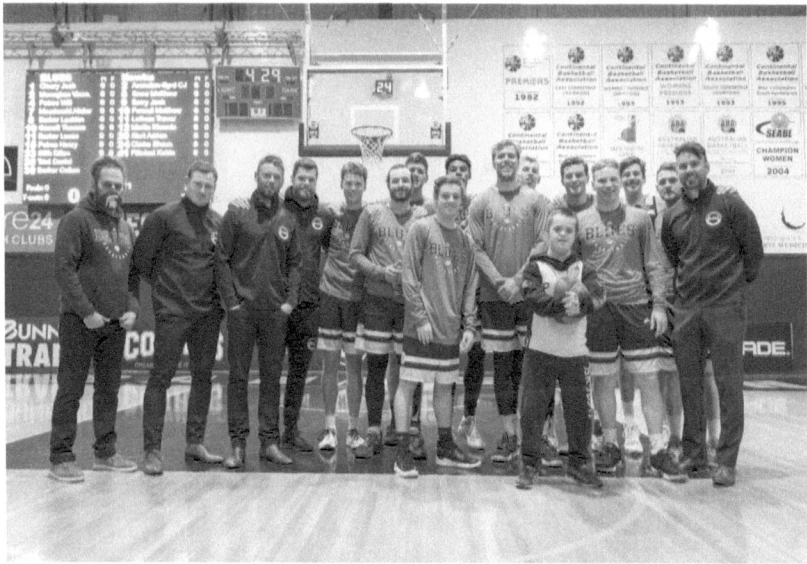

Frankston Blues Basketball – creating an amazing inclusive area with many new opportunities for people of all abilities.

You know the child that sits by themselves?
Go sit with them.

You know the child who always eats alone in the yard?
Go eat with them.

You know the child that sits at the back of the classroom alone?
Go talk to them.

You never know the impacts a small gesture will have on a child.

FIM
Friend in Me
Original Author - Unknown

WHAT PEOPLE ARE SAYING

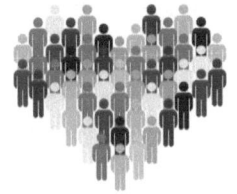

Can you imagine a world where everybody truly accepted one another? This is just the start of that conversation for some, and the continued fight for others like Julie and Darcy. Thank you so much to the both of you for sharing your story and lived experience when it comes to this massively important topic. I know firsthand that it hasn't been easy at times, but I also know that it's been because of those challenges that you continue to advocate for real acceptance and inclusion. This book is an important step in the right direction, and I genuinely cannot wait for people to start reading.

KRISTIAN SERAINIDIS
Founder, PROJECT KICK IT

It seems wrong that people need to be told that everyone has the right to feel included and accepted: it should be instinctual. We all know that being excluded hurts. Julie speaks from the heart about her experience of exclusion and inclusion in an engaging way that cuts through the noise. She shows us that our actions and words can and do have an impact on others, giving us a raw insight into how this feels. She also shares advice for those who have experienced exclusion firsthand, encouraging them to not hide away, but to get out and live life to the fullest. Amazing stuff Julie. Your words really resonated with me and I'm so pleased you have written this book. I feel inspired to do better, as I'm sure others will too.

MARINDA WILKINSON
Copywriter & Editor, Vivid Words

I had the good fortune to meet Julie at a Carers Victoria 'Mingle' event for family carers. Here was this positive, confident, mother of four standing in front of me telling me about her first book, *The Unexpected Journey*, which describes her DS journey with youngest child, Darcy and the wonderful care he receives from his family. One of the most important things I've learned while working at Carers Victoria is that carers trust other carers. By entering into the world of writing and now with a second book to her name, Julie is generously imparting the many life lessons she has learned about caring for Darcy, so other carers can feel more confident about initially stepping into a world of the unknown. Julie's lived experience is a lifeline for so many other carers and she is to be congratulated for her honesty and transparency sharing her journey through writing and making so many people's lives better.

ANNIE HAYWARD
GM Policy Strategy & Public Affairs,
Carers Victoria, 2015–2020.

The Unexpected Journey is a relatable, emotive and powerful story shared through the lived experience of a courageous mother and woman. Julie's ability to capture and articulate Darcy and her family's journey will resonate with all parents, as well as provide a few laughs and tears along the way. Every individual brings diverse abilities and attributes which make our world a better place and Julie expresses this beautifully throughout her writing. In this, her second book, Julie shares personal stories of the profound impact of inclusion, and why it is critically important as a society we provide equal access to opportunities and resources for people who might otherwise be excluded or marginalised. Congratulations Julie on sharing your story which has many more exciting chapters to come!

DAN PAYNE
CEO, Down Syndrome Victoria

Congratulations Julie, on so many fronts. For the positive outlook you maintained through every challenge, and for all the fun and love you have with your beautiful boy.

The Unexpected Journey is an inspiring read on what matters most and on finding joy in the challenge, and moving through acceptance, inclusion and love. Go Julie and go Darcy!

GREG PLANT
Director, Powerplant

When I began reading Julie's first book, *The Unexpected Journey*, it was really hard to put down. Eloquent and easy to read, just like listening to Julie speak. Although I have never met Darcy, I now feel like I know him to some degree.

I'm in awe of Julie's positive attitude, and the beautiful people who support her. You can certainly see how her life has been enriched, not stifled, by disability. Julie is just a mum, like us all, but perhaps with more energy! She is the epitome of a loving mother, wanting nothing but the best for all her children. Strong enough to make the right decisions for her family, she takes on board the professionals' information and advice, but at times, chooses to make their journey their own. Julie is not afraid to stand up and be heard. There are lessons to be learnt here, which I find humbling and somewhat liberating.

Julie has shown us that DS is not the stigma that society makes it out to be. Yes, it is a disability and not the 'norm', but there is absolutely no reason why the lives of people living with DS should be any different than our own. They are real, have feelings, dreams and goals ... and although it may take a bit longer to achieve, they can get there. They are super caring and super happy individuals that have the ability, like all of us, to contribute to society.

Julie has given us more than a book – it is a valuable resource that will certainly be helpful for future DS families, and for medical professionals to recommend. Doctors may have the scientific facts, but they don't have the actual experience. And for those of us not on that journey with disability, it is an eye-opener that gives us an insight that perhaps we may have never realised. *The Magic of Inclusion* is a book that everyone should read to understand why this is so important and why nobody should be made to feel excluded from anything in life.

MONICA STABLES
Colleague, Berettas Langwarrin

If you're looking for confirmation that you're not alone in this, then *The Unexpected Journey* is a must read. Rest assured Julie's books will make you feel at ease, uplifted and will leave you with a general sense of I can do this.

Get on board, you won't regret it!

TRACEY McCARTNEY

CONTENTS

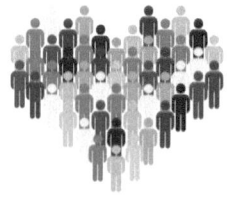

WHAT PEOPLE ARE SAYING	7
DEDICATION	15
THANK YOU	17
MY SON	21
INTRODUCTION	25
REFLECTION	29
FOREWORD	33
CHAPTER 1: IN THIS TOGETHER	35
CHAPTER 2: EMPOWERING OPPORTUNITIES	43
CHAPTER 3: EMBRACING ABILITY	55
CHAPTER 4: THE INCLUSION SUPERPOWER	63
CHAPTER 5: GROWING STRONG TOGETHER	73
CHAPTER 6: WE MUST DO BETTER	79
CHAPTER 7: SEEING THE GREATNESS	89
CHAPTER 8: A PLACE TO SHINE	97

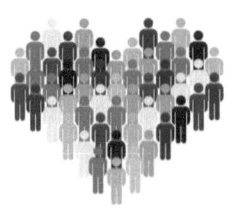

CHAPTER 9: GETTING THERE, DOING THAT!	105
CHAPTER 10: TOGETHER WE STAND	113
CHAPTER 11: SPEAK NO EVIL	117
CHAPTER 12: WE CAN, SO WE MUST!	127
CHAPTER 13: OUR AMAZING BOY	133
CHAPTER 14: FINAL THOUGHTS	143
FROM THE HEARTS AND MINDS OF MUMS	147
AHA MOMENTS AND TAKEAWAYS	161
AFTERWORD	163
ABOUT THE AUTHOR	167
ACKNOWLEDGEMENTS	169
OFFERS	171
LINKS FOR SUPPORT SERVICES AND ORGANISATIONS THAT PROMOTE INCLUSION THAT WE HAVE USED AND ARE PART OF	177

DEDICATION

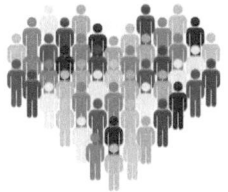

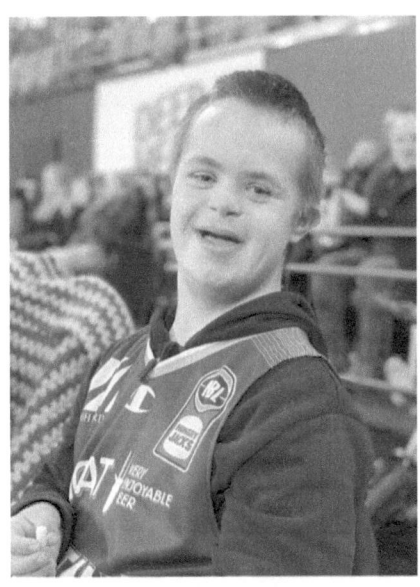

I dedicate this book to my son Darcy. He is an amazing boy who lives with Down Syndrome. He teaches me lessons every single day. He has taught me to think outside the box and not worry about what other people think. If you want to do something, there is always a way this can happen. His love for life and all he enjoys is infectious and wonderful to be around.

He enjoys everything he does as though it's the first time he has done it.

We wouldn't change Darcy for the world, but we are changing the world for Darcy.

Thank you, my beautiful boy, for choosing us as your family ... we are truly blessed.

THANK YOU

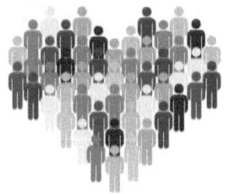

Thank you to my family Mick, Caleb, Blake, Darcy and our beautiful gypsy girl Bree. The support you show me each and every day is something I cherish and has helped me pursue my dreams. I love you all with all my heart and you are all my WHY. Why I want to be successful in my future dreams and passions.

Thank you to my friends who have also supported me 100%. You help me to keep going even when I sometimes feel like there's no point. You give me guidance and love and help me to keep on track.

My mentors, friends and employers at Ultimate 48 Hour Author. Thank you for giving me the tools and support to help me achieve my dream of writing books, and the confidence to expand on those books to help other people. It is so inspiring and motivational to assist at your events and be part of the team. I am so lucky and very grateful to have you all in my life and I hope I make you proud.

THE MAGIC OF INCLUSION

Trudi Paydon, you are our angel and such a huge part of our family. You taught me it is okay to fight for what is right and what I believe in. You fought for our boy's inclusion and look where he is today. Without you and your support, I do not know how we would have made it through those primary years. You and Darcy are amazing.

Caroline, you are a very important part of our family and we cherish that you continue to do all the wonderful things with Darcy that we have always done. Putting him forward and showing the world how amazing he is. You are Darcy's favourite and he often pretend calls you to dob on us for various things … so funny. Having Jake in our life now is also amazing, as Darcy has gained a third brother and a best friend. We love you and are so grateful to have you in our lives.

Kristian and Emma from Project KICK IT. We met you guys in lockdown, and it's been a blast ever since. What you have created with the awesome experiences for our kids is the best. The experiences, the independence they feel just doing life with a group of their friends is amazing. Darcy loves hanging out with you (so do we), and we are so happy to be part of your lives.

THANK YOU

There is only one way to look at things, until someone shows us how to look at them with different eyes.

PABLO PICASSO

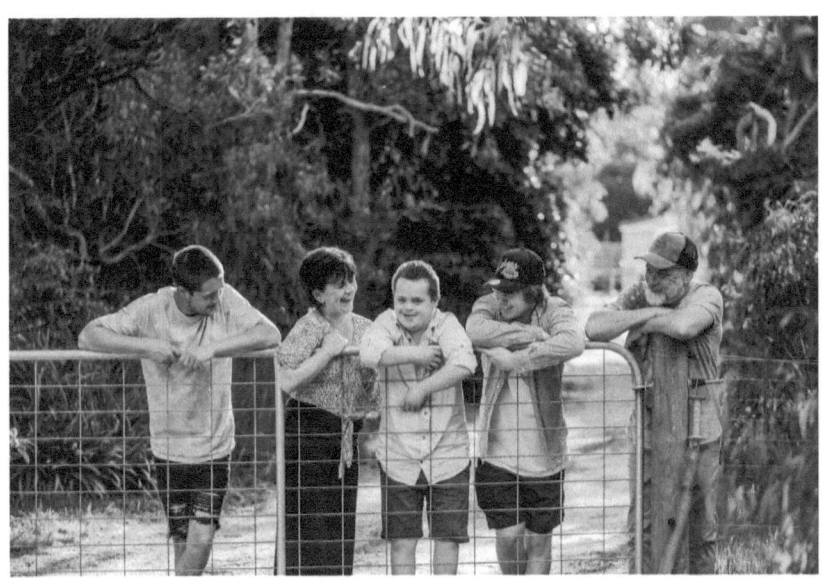

MY SON

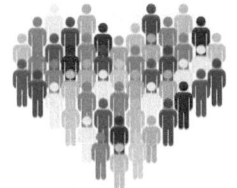

My children are my everything and I love them all equally with all my heart and everything I have inside of me. I will protect them any way I can and do whatever I can to guide them and be by their side.

My son Darcy however, has some wonderful qualities that stand him out from the crowd.

He does have Down Syndrome, but that is not it. That is merely a part of him.

He is the reason I fulfilled my dream of becoming an author and he is the reason my journey is going further to advocate for him and others like him, to show people how wonderful the world of disability can be, to help other families and to show everyone how important inclusion is.

My older children have the same dreams for their younger brother and want him to be accepted so he can enjoy everything they have enjoyed.

One of the most wonderful qualities Darcy has is no judgement toward others. This is a quality I think we should all take something from and learn from.

He takes people for who they are, not what they have, what they look like or what they can and cannot do.

I love this about him.

He also has this amazing quality of seeing things like he is seeing them for the first time and truly embraces every experience.

Everything he experiences is wonderful. He embraces what is there and relishes in the positives about what he is doing.

I think we can all learn from people like Darcy and his friends.

Learn to see the person, not the disability.

Learn to give people a chance.

Learn to be non-judgemental and take people for how you find them and who they are.

He has taught us these beautiful things and I hope others can also learn the same.

MY SON

Inclusion is not bringing people into what already exists, it is making a new space, a better space for everyone.

GEORGE DEI

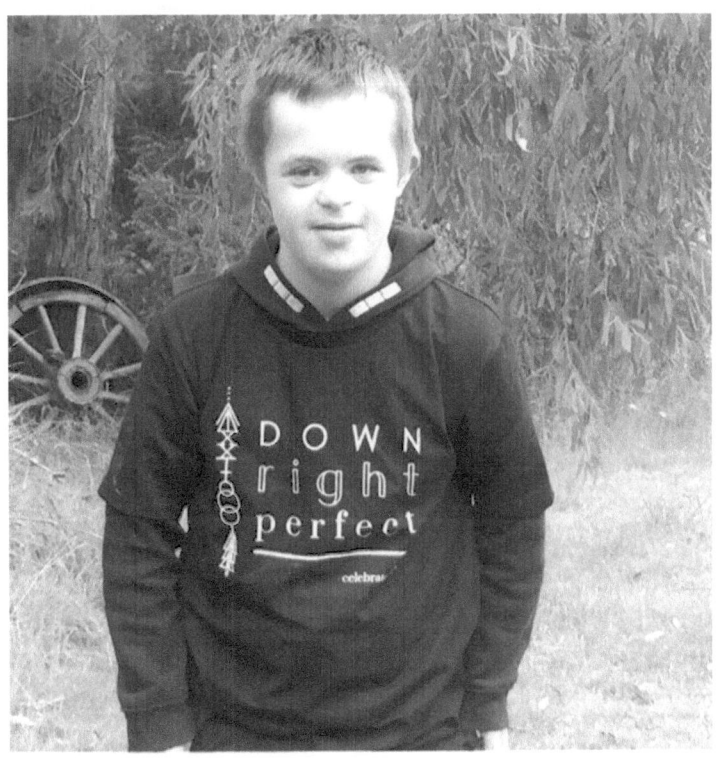

INTRODUCTION

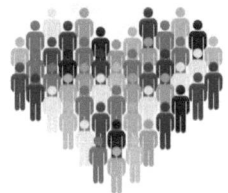

My dream of writing a book became a reality with *The Unexpected Journey: Embracing the Beauty of Disability.*

Becoming an author was so much more than I had imagined. The people I have become friends with because of the process has been amazing. These people are inspiring and extremely motivational. They give me guidance every day.

The experience of publishing my first book opened my mind to a whole new world of where I wanted to be and what I wanted to be doing. It also inspired me to keep writing.

Sharing our story and letting people into the amazing world we are part of has been something far more wonderful that I could have ever imagined. Showing people Darcy is capable of anything that anyone else is and showing people it's alright to give people a chance is one of the big reasons I think it is important to share our experiences. To show people that everyone deserves a chance.

After completing my first book, I soon found myself raising awareness on many platforms and becoming an advocate for people with disabilities, and everyone who feels they are a little different. I hope that I represent them well, and I hope I teach people to embrace difference, and not be scared of it.

Two of my favourite sayings are, 'Look at the person, not the disability' and 'Ability not disability'.

The Magic of Inclusion: Give People a Chance and Watch Them Shine is a book about acceptance and inclusion from a mum's point of view. It includes real-life experiences of families living with disability, and shares simple but powerful ways in how we can all make these two words, acceptance and inclusion, something that happens all the time. They do go hand in hand … without acceptance you can't include. You have to open up your mind and see the person and understand they have the right to participate in all types of activities, just like anybody else.

In raising awareness that actions and words can be cruel, I have found many people don't even realise they are making someone feel uncomfortable in a situation. It's important for them to know. Changing the way someone says something and the way they interact with someone can make a world of difference.

The Magic of Inclusion is a term I love because we all have the power to make inclusion happen and see the magic that happens. And inclusion and acceptance isn't a topic that should be talked about just in disability. My experiences are from what we have dealt with and what I have watched my friends deal with, but it can happen anywhere, and to anyone.

INTRODUCTION

With this book, I hope to help more people to embrace difference – and in doing so, help more people to feel confident to go out and enjoy life, just like everybody else. To be free to participate in sport, schooling, work and all the other everyday things a lot of us take for granted because we can just access it whenever we like.

Some people need a little assistance to be able to participate in activities, but once you give them the help, guidance, resources, and a chance to have a go, you will be amazed at the result. Some people just lack confidence, so opening up your heart and showing them it's okay, is just a small step you can take to make someone feel included.

I hope my book helps people to step out and assist others where they need it. We all need help from time to time. Even without a disability, sometimes a little help and kindness goes a long way.

Enjoy this book, take some lessons from it and use them to the best of your ability.

Thank you Darcy, for choosing us and thank you for teaching us every day.

Diversity is a fact, inclusion is an act.
AUTHOR UNKNOWN

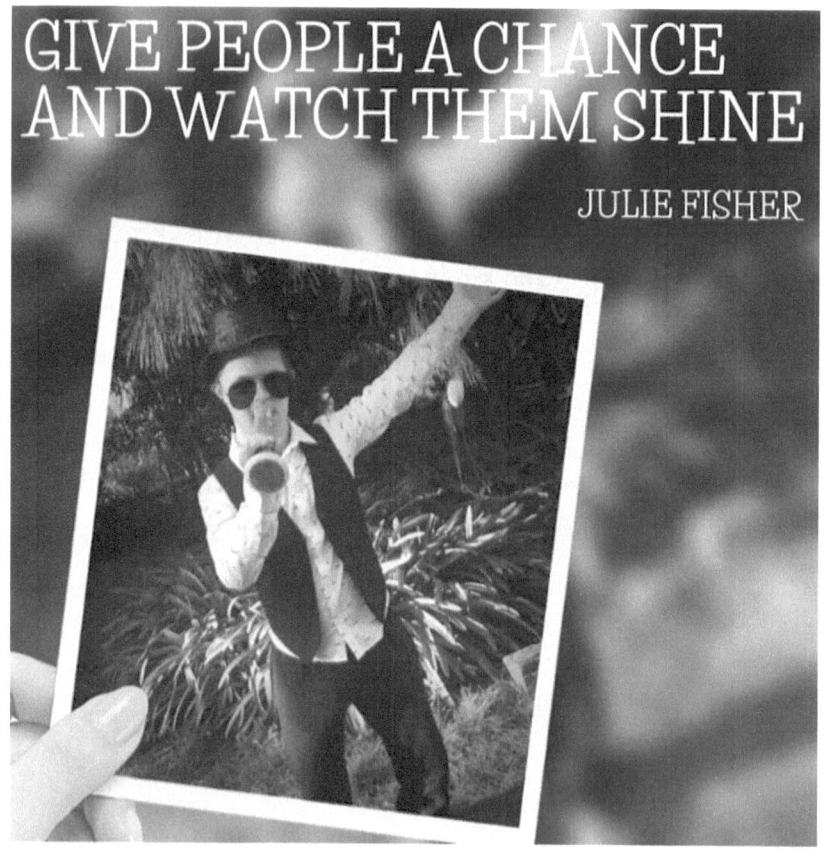

REFLECTION

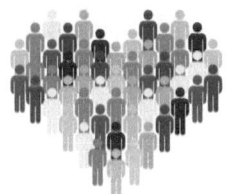

When we start a family, we see the future with our children as happy and bright, with them doing all the things they wish. We work towards making sure we have the time and capabilities to make their dreams come true and give them every chance possible for a bright future.

It is no different when you have a child with special or additional needs. You still plan to do whatever is possible to make sure they can achieve their dreams and build toward a bright future. We want our children to grow, and we encourage whatever direction they choose to take. We want our children to have a successful and happy life.

When we discovered our son Darcy had Down Syndrome, I immediately started to focus on goals and supports he would need.

We were lucky because we had an army of support that guided us toward the early intervention we needed to make sure he had a good start. Support platforms, in my mind, are extremely important. It is good to be around like-minded people because they know exactly what you are going through and have many valuable resources and answers to questions you may have.

The thing we weren't ready for, as he got older and started wanting to participate in the same sports as his brothers and with his dual schooling, was the barriers we came across and the campaigning we had to do to make sure he could at least have a chance to give things a try.

We weren't ready for people to question whether he could do what he wanted to do. They questioned whether he would be up to it when we wanted him to attend mainstream camp. This really put a dampener on what we were looking forward to as a wonderful time for our son. Once we advocated for him and he was given a chance, they were amazed at how well he did.

One question we asked was … do you think we would put him forward if we didn't think he could do it?

The advocating and campaigning is becoming less and less as the world starts to see people of all-abilities just as able as anyone else. Social media, for example, can be a platform where people can see that anyone can shine.

The Magic of Inclusion is about how important inclusion and acceptance is and how easy it is to help people accomplish their goals. There is something out there for everyone.

Everyone has different abilities and everyone needs different supports. From watching my friends with children with various additional needs, I have seen that many things are possible. With love, kindness,

REFLECTION

some support and focusing on what they enjoy, we can make things happen for them.

When Darcy was younger, we didn't know when he would walk or when he may become verbal, and we were not sure of what other things he may or may not be able to do. As he grew, even though these milestones of walking and talking took some time, he did succeed. We still work very closely with him to work on goals, but with time, patience and love, we will see him reach those goals we are setting for him.

Everyone's goals and dreams are different, and by giving people a chance, no matter what they are able to accomplish, really does help tremendously.

Sometimes you have to just think outside the box a little. When you do this, you will be amazed at the results that come with it.

> Sometimes the greatest gift you can give another is to simply include them.
> **AUTHOR UNKNOWN**

FOREWORD

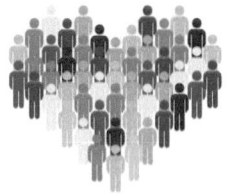

Julie Fisher is a gift to the world, and she doesn't even know it.

She enlightens us with her selfless attitude and her mission to spread awareness across the globe for people living with a disability, in particular, Down Syndrome.

My name is Louise Larkin, and I am the founder of Friend In Me. I am on a mission to make social inclusion a priority and to make sure that no child is left behind. Not today. Not tomorrow. Not ever.

I connected with Julie through the big world of social media after hearing about her being an inspirational author and a fierce advocate for her son Darcy who was born with Down Syndrome.

Julie's second book *The Magic of Inclusion* is an absolute treasure to parents, teachers and caregivers to teach the power of inclusion.

Her tagline 'Give people a chance and watch them shine' is something that I very strongly live by with our work through Friend in Me, but it is also such a strong message that needs to be spread across the globe.

Imagine the world with more people like Julie …

Imagine the world with everyone advocating to give people living with disability a chance.

Imagine a world that was full of inclusion … imagine how beautiful that would be.

Julie, thank you for being the voice when others cannot be heard.

Thank you for spreading the awareness in dedication of your beautiful boy Darcy and his community.

Thank you for being you.

LOUISE LARKIN
Founder & Chief Inclusion Officer
Friend In Me

CHAPTER 1

IN THIS TOGETHER

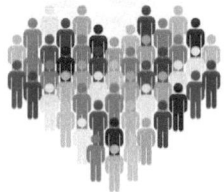

Diversity is inviting new people to the party, inclusion is asking them to dance.

VERNA MYERS

Before I begin, the most important piece of advice I can give all of you is, when you are involved with or see someone with a disability you need to ...

'SEE THE PERSON FIRST AND FOREMOST'

Their disability is just something they live with. They have the same needs and wants as everyone else.

THE MAGIC OF INCLUSION

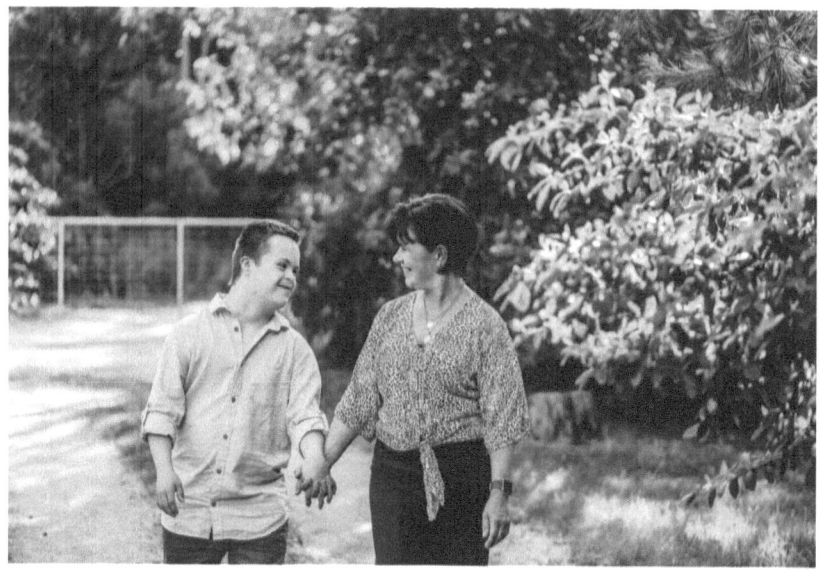

Acceptance and inclusion are pretty easy words to understand. Most people would like to think they are accepting of all people around them and would include them in any activities they may be doing. I think a lot of people would be quite upset and shocked if they thought they weren't accepting of other people. Sometimes I don't think we realise that we are making people feel like they shouldn't be there. A simple act of staring at someone can make them, or the person they are with, feel like there is something wrong with them, which immediately makes them feel as though they are not accepted. You may not even realise you are doing it.

As a mum of a young teenage boy with Down Syndrome, I find that acceptance and inclusion isn't as forthcoming as we would like to think. People look at my son's disability before they do anything else, and immediately assume he is unable to participate or understand what they are saying.

IN THIS TOGETHER

I remember being taught at a very young age to never assume and to never judge people, especially if you haven't even seen what they are capable of.

I don't think people realise that the person they are excluding actually does know what is going on. They DO understand. Even if they can't verbalise how they are feeling, they know exactly what is going on.

Imagine how you would feel if people excluded you from something just because of the way you looked or because of some of your behavioural traits. Have you ever thought about that? Because that is exactly what is happening.

My son Darcy gets upset and doesn't understand why he may feel as though he is not being allowed to do something, or even be given a chance to have a go. This happens when people are staring and being judgemental, and it's very difficult for me to explain to him. He is aware of what is going on.

One of the things I do when we are about to start something new, especially if it is a sporting program, is to talk to the person in charge and explain that he may need a little extra coaching and maybe a little bit of one on one. But once he gets it, the SKY IS THE LIMIT.

We have done this several times, but Auskick was the sport that it was really implemented. We attended our local clinic as the all-abilities Auskick he had been attending was not running anymore. It was great because it was just other parents running the clinic and doing the coaching and they were very easy to approach and talk to. Once they knew I was also more than approachable, they asked what needed to be done (if anything) and away they went with him.

His skills in football are fantastic and that's because people gave him a chance instead of looking at him and deciding it wouldn't work.

> '***Inclusion*** *means that all people, regardless of their abilities, disabilities, or health care needs, have the right to: Be respected and appreciated as valuable members of their communities. Participate in recreational activities in neighbourhood settings.*'
>
> Institute for Community Inclusion, 'What we mean when we talk about inclusion', ICI, no date.

Inclusion can come in many different forms. At times, all you may have to do is actually accept the person into the group and that's it. Other times, you may have to do a little extra to make sure they understand how to do something. Some people may need visual assistance, others might need instructions one at a time. Small changes such as these are often all it takes to make sure everyone is able to process the information properly.

In any event, I don't think it's such a huge ask to just give someone a chance, and the extra steps or strategies that may need to be put in place would not take up a lot of time. Giving instructions one step at a time is not difficult to put in place, but it can make all the difference for someone.

Acceptance is exactly the same. People with disabilities have the same emotions and feelings as everyone else. They want to be loved, liked and have friends. They want to experience all the same things everyone else does. They want to learn, and they want to embrace life to the fullest.

WE ALL HAVE THE SAME NEEDS AND WANTS.

IN THIS TOGETHER

And again, if you just give someone a chance, I guarantee you will be amazed. It's really not that hard just to be kind.

Sometimes people stare at others without even realising what they're doing. I know I have stared at people only because I like to watch people. I find them fascinating. When I realise what I am doing, I immediately smile so they know I'm not looking at them in a negative way and try to make the situation not too awkward.

But since having Darcy, I've realised that staring at people is actually very uncomfortable for them and I had never thought about that before. You may not be staring at them in a negative way, but because it is a stare, it feels negative. It makes people feel like there is something wrong with them.

People also talk to me instead of Darcy. This indicates that they think he has no idea or understanding of what they are saying. Speaking to me instead of him makes him feel like he is not as accepted as everyone else.

A simple thing like talking to my son, instead of me, is a HUGE step toward acceptance. He may not be able to answer questions as clearly as me, but he understands what is being said and can communicate even with a visual answer by him showing you.

I have a friend with a daughter who is non-verbal, but when she is being spoken to, you can see she understands as she communicates with her eyes. You know exactly how she is feeling just by the way she is looking at you.

In our local community, my son is accepted and has quite a following of people that want to know how he is and what he is doing.

They love seeing him out and about with me and watching how much he is growing and thriving, and they love to see what he is accomplishing.

I am very comfortable taking him to our local community shopping centre because I know we will not encounter remarks, stares and pointing. Everyone we see there, gives him a smile and a wave and he loves to visit all the shop owners and say hello. They all look more than happy when they see him come through the door because he brings a very positive and happy vibe with him. He loves to say hello and see what is happening.

Just one suburb away, at a slightly larger shopping complex, the acceptance is not there. I find myself guarding him as we walk around looking at the shops. I do this I think because I don't want him to see some of the stares and pointing that happens and I don't want him to feel uncomfortable. I want him to be happy being in any place we go, just as he is in our own local shopping centre.

We all deserve to feel welcomed and accepted in our surroundings. Imagine going somewhere knowing that people were going to stare, point and talk about you because you are a little different in their eyes. Imagine the anxiety building up in someone knowing this is going to happen when they enter a shopping centre, movies, park or anywhere else they may go.

The anxiety builds up so much, they end up not wanting to go anywhere. Just staying home feeling like they have no friends or anyone to enjoy things with. This anxiety also exists in the parents of these children. They too end up feeling like they can't take their children anywhere because of how people are making them feel.

IN THIS TOGETHER

Put yourself and your children in my shoes and in Darcy's. Imagine taking your child out and feeling like everyone is staring and pointing at them for no reason apart from the fact that they look a little different, speak a little different or anything similar to this.

This happened to us just the other day. We went to a shopping centre, and as we entered, a young man nudged his friend and pointed at Darcy as though to say, 'look at him'. I really don't understand the need to do this. What benefit does it have for anyone? It just makes us feel uncomfortable.

How do you think you would cope with that? How would you feel if most places you went to, you were made to feel as though your child isn't worthy of being there? Because that is what it feels like.

Instead of staring without any emotion, when someone sees you looking at them, a simple act of smiling changes everything.

It makes people feel happy because someone is acknowledging them instead of just looking at them.

It gives them confidence instead of anxiety.

It makes them feel like they belong.

Now go forth and be kind, be grateful and be inclusive.

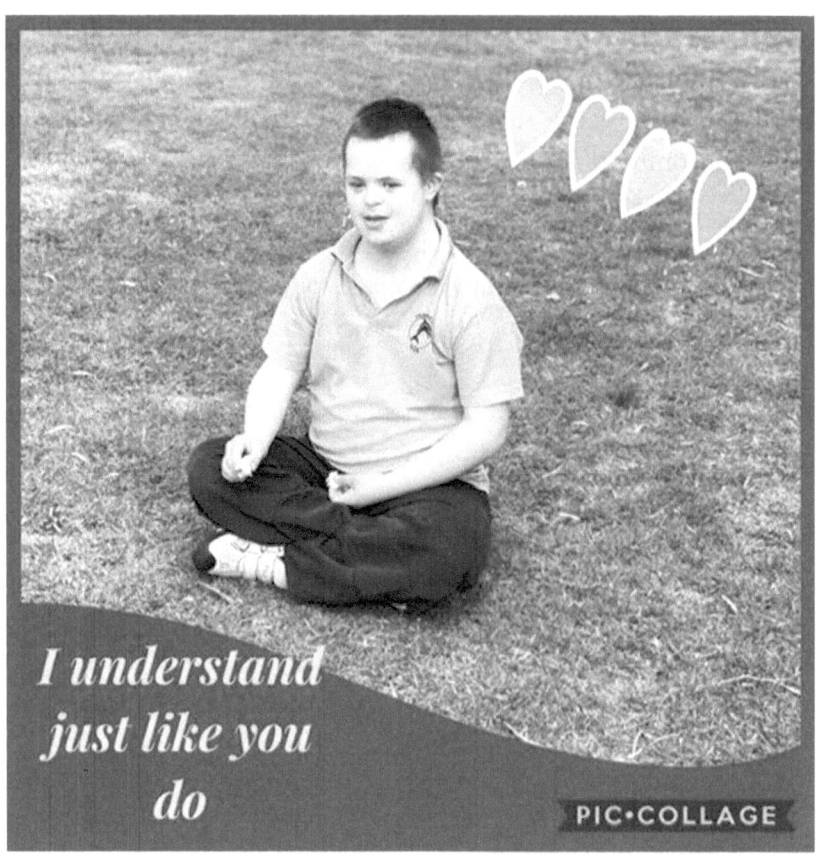

CHAPTER 2

EMPOWERING OPPORTUNITIES

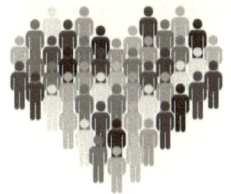

> When everyone is included, everyone wins.
> **JESSE JACKSON**

I suppose most people would wonder why they need to bother knowing about inclusion because they probably think it will never affect them.

WRONG!!!!!!

Even if you do not experience the negativity of exclusion personally, there are people everywhere around you that do experience it. It happens to so many people every day and it is not just limited to people living with a disability. Many people feel as though they are not being accepted and included.

I am writing this book based on my experience with having a son that lives with Down Syndrome, but as I said above, exclusion happens to so many every day. You may be at your local shop, or the beach or park and it may be happening right in front of you to someone else.

This is where it is okay to stand up and give a hand to others, to show that it is alright to give them a chance. You don't have to make a scene by pointing out someone specifically, but you could just walk past and say hello or smile. A small gesture like this can often be enough to make the negativity disappear.

Teach your children to not be afraid of someone just because they look a little different or behave differently to what they are used to. Teach them how to help out instead of just stand and stare and make remarks.

Sometimes, someone else's child may be quite anxious about where they are or what they are about to do. Sometimes it is because of the reaction of others that they feel this way.

So, be inclusive and help the other parent out a little. Also help the person that is being made to feel left out. Go over and offer some assistance. Say to the child, it is okay. Have a try and if you need help, we will all help you.

The sense of accomplishment when the child has actually given it a go will fill your heart with such joy and pride. And even if they don't get

EMPOWERING OPPORTUNITIES

it 100% right the first time, just having the chance to learn gives them the confidence to have another go and keep on going. It is amazing to watch someone feel accomplished. It is the best feeling on this earth.

It will also make the parent or carer feel very supported and not singled out amongst the crowd. This is extremely important because it is the parent that is bringing the child to the activity. If they feel as though their child is not being given a chance and being accepted, they will not take them again. I know this because I have felt it firsthand, and I have friends that have felt this also.

Sometimes even just going to the shopping centre can be very overwhelming when you are waiting and worrying about people's reactions. The anxiety builds up tremendously. Just being kind and thinking about how your reactions may make someone feel, will help them feel relaxed about taking their child out, even to the shops.

The feeling you get when everyone is looking, and pointing is overwhelming and not a nice feeling. We pretend it doesn't matter and soldier on by taking our child by the hand and going somewhere else.

BUT IT DOES MATTER!!!

Why should any parent feel singled out just because they want their child to experience things any other child does? They have as much right as anybody else. They're not hurting anyone or doing anything nasty, so why should they be excluded? Just because they look and sometimes behave a little different? Because sometimes they may need a little extra assistance? Not good excuses to exclude anybody in my opinion.

I will give you an example of something that happened to me and Darcy when he was just 18 months old …

THE MAGIC OF INCLUSION

We joined a local music group. I thought it would be amazing and would help Darcy with some of his social skills as well as fine motor skills. I also thought it would be great to meet some other mums and be part of something Darcy really loved – music.

I will admit that as soon as we entered the room, there were two ladies that made me feel uncomfortable. I brushed it off and decided it was just me being sensitive.

We had been going for about four weeks when the teacher started a new activity. We were all to get into a circle with an instrument and as the music went on, we would swap instruments with the person to our left.

The activity was wonderful and very engaging. Darcy really loved passing his instrument to the next person and receiving a different one to try.

As it went on, one of the ladies I felt uncomfortable with was to swap instruments with us. She looked at me, looked at Darcy and walked around us to the next person.

My heart absolutely sunk and began to ache. I wanted to scream at her and cry at the same time. What was wrong with Darcy? Why did she do that?

I pretended like nothing had happened and then the next lady I felt uncomfortable with did the same thing.

WHAT IS GOING ON? I wanted to crawl into a big hole because I felt so sad.

EMPOWERING OPPORTUNITIES

We finished the activity, I packed up our things and left. We never went back. I decided I didn't want Darcy being around people like that and I definitely didn't want him being treated like that.

I did contact the lady running the program, told her what had happened and that we would not be returning. She was very disappointed and embarrassed, and wanted us to return, but I told her I would not put my son in the same company as people like that. He did not deserve to be treated like that.

It doesn't take much to make someone feel part of the group. Those ladies I've just talked about only had to pass an instrument to Darcy and take the one he was giving to them. They didn't have to do anything else. All they had to do was smile and continue with the activity. Everyone would have felt happy with this. Being kind helps others feel accepted. It makes them feel welcome, so that they want to be part of the group or take part in the activity.

When somebody feels like they are accepted and included don't you think it would make them want to try a little harder, to feel relaxed enough to give it a go? I think it does 100%.

> '**Inclusion** is seen as a universal human right. The **aim of inclusion** is to embrace all people irrespective of race, gender, disability, medical or other need. It is about giving equal access and opportunities and getting rid of discrimination and intolerance (removal of barriers). It affects all aspects of public life.'
>
> Inclusion.Me, 'What does inclusion mean?', *Inclusion.Me Ltd.*, 17 January 2008.

THE MAGIC OF INCLUSION

I have seen firsthand what it does to a child and the children around them when they are publicly excluded. As an adult, it is very hard trying to explain to children why their friend cannot do what they are doing. It is actually heartbreaking when all they want to do is play or participate in an activity just like everyone else.

Imagine yourself going to the movies, or even just out shopping, and when you arrive people stop and stare at you or move out of the way like you have something they will catch. Imagine your child being the only one who is never invited to a birthday party. How would that make you feel? It may just be because you look a little different, walk a little differently or something else, but whatever it is, when people do this, it makes you feel like you shouldn't be there, when in fact, you have just as much right as anybody else.

If you can't imagine how it feels, then put yourself into the shoes of others and think about how it may make you feel. Try to imagine how you would feel if people made you feel like you shouldn't be there.

Think about if you walk into a shop to make a purchase. You walk in, smile at the people in the shop, and instead of them returning the smile, they look at you strangely and move out of the way. How would that make you feel?

With my son Darcy, when people stare or move out of the way, (and believe me, it has happened), as I have said earlier, I try to smile or say hello. Just so it isn't negative for him. Inside I am breaking and sometimes getting quite angry, but on the outside, I have to make him feel okay.

Sometimes, I'm not very good at not responding. Just the other day when I was with Darcy at the supermarket, a lady was heading towards us with her son. As she approached us, she took her son by the arm and moved him away so he wouldn't walk past Darcy. I couldn't contain myself this particular day and told her 'It's okay, he won't catch anything'. It makes me mad, and I really don't understand behaviour like this.

At 15, he knows what is going on. He understands negativity and exclusion and I can see he doesn't like how it feels. When he feels like this, he moves closer to me and buries his head into my side. He holds onto my arm and puts his head down. I hate it when he feels like this.

Just by being kind and positive to others by smiling or saying hello, I find that by the time we get home, I don't feel so bad. We have been out and ended up having a good day, so I don't hold onto it. It has taken me a long time to get to this point because really, all I want to do is ask them what their problem is and why they are staring or pointing at my son.

When I respond in a negative way by commenting on their behaviour, I find that I hold onto it for a long time. It's hard not to respond sometimes.

It is quite different and harder to deal with when someone makes a passing comment. I try not to hold onto it, but I do, and it stays with you. It stays because you don't understand why people have to say anything at all. It isn't their child, and they don't have to look after them, so why make a negative comment? Does it make them feel better? Do they feel accomplished by doing so? Because it doesn't make the person they are commenting about or who they are with feel good at all.

I have comments that have been made over the years still in my head and my heart and some of these were made years ago. I remember them like they just happened.

THE MAGIC OF INCLUSION

How would you feel if someone made a negative comment about your child just because of something they are doing, something they are wearing or the fact that they may not speak clearly? I will tell you how you would feel: NOT GOOD AT ALL.

One of the things that happened to us, and stands out very clearly in my mind to this day was when we were waiting to be picked up by a friend from the movies …

> *Darcy and I were at the movies one time and were waiting out the front to be picked up by a friend. We'd had a wonderful day and the movie was great. We both really enjoyed it and were thoroughly enjoying our day.*
>
> *At the time, Darcy was about 10 or 11 and he was incontinent. So, he had pull ups on. No big deal and something that doesn't affect anybody else.*
>
> *As we were waiting for our friend to pick us up, Darcy was bent over looking at the stars on the concrete. A lady walked past with her son who, at a guess, was around 12.*
>
> *As she walked past, she looked at Darcy and then turned to her son and said, 'Ugh! He's wearing a nappy! How disgusting'.*
>
> *Now what in the actual hell was that??!!!! What business was it of hers for a start that Darcy wore pull ups and what difference did it make to her life? Why did she say this to her son? What was that teaching him?*
>
> *This woman was very lucky, because I actually couldn't believe my ears and it took a few minutes for me to register what she had said. By the time I was ready to react, she was long gone.*

EMPOWERING OPPORTUNITIES

If I had of reacted immediately, she wouldn't have liked what I had to say to her, and it would have probably ended up being a very awful experience.

Please don't ever be like this lady. Her comments made a great day turn into an awful day where I went home very upset and confused at why she had made those remarks. The only thing I was thankful for was that Darcy didn't hear her.

So just always remember, that **everyone is different**, but everyone is also the same. We all have the same feelings and wants in life.

Please remember that. You don't have to engage with and be friends with everyone, but negative acts and comments hurt. Instead of staring, give a smile. It is a small but positive act that goes a long way in helping that person have the confidence to keep going with what they are doing.

Before you make a comment that may be rude toward someone, like the lady I just mentioned, think before you speak. Don't say anything at all. Especially in front of the mother of the child you are talking about, and also in front of the child.

I often hear people referring to others as 'not normal' and if I can, I usually always make a comment because of a lovely man I once met many years ago. He told me about his disability and how he had an accident. He said he hears people talk about others not being normal and he always responds with this …

What is normal? I'll tell you what normal is. It's a setting on a washing machine.

I have never forgotten this, and I refer to it regularly. I never saw that man again, but I think about him a lot and wonder how he is going. I'm glad we spoke and I'm glad he told me about his answer to normal.

When I say include, you don't have to physically do anything to make sure this happens. Just by being friendly, kind and giving a positive vibe, you will help the person to feel like it is alright for them to be there and have a go. When you do this, you are definitely helping to make someone feel much more confident being where they are. I think this is something we can all do to include others.

We need to make sure everyone has a chance to participate and shine. When you give people a chance, you will be amazed at what they can achieve and how easily they can participate in all the activities that everyone does.

I think every child deserves to feel comfortable going to the movies, eating out, going to the park, going to the beach or swimming pool, playing games, going shopping or whatever else they may want to do. Everyone deserves the chance to experience things.

Including also gives their parent or carer much more confidence in taking them places. Sometimes the inclusive behaviour is more beneficial for them, because they are the ones taking them out. I have seen parents diminish in confidence with taking their child out because of how other people make them feel. This is WRONG! Nobody should be made to feel as though they shouldn't take their child anywhere.

Again, imagine if you felt like you couldn't take your child out to a movie, or to the circus or a carnival, the park, the beach and the list goes on. Imagine not having the confidence to take them anywhere. All because of how a stranger may have made you feel. You wouldn't like it.

EMPOWERING OPPORTUNITIES

So if you're wondering 'why include?', it is because everyone, including parents and carers, as well as the child or person they are looking after, deserves a chance to experience life and experience all of the wonderful things they want to take part in.

CHAPTER 3

EMBRACING ABILITY

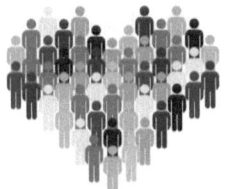

Inclusion is not simply about physical proximity. It is about intentionally planning for the success of all students.

THINK INCLUSIVE

As I mentioned in the previous chapter, we need inclusion because nobody should ever be made to feel like they don't belong. We should have the opportunity to show everyone around us, and the world, how capable we can be. And also, to show that it is okay to embrace difference. After all, we are all different in many ways.

THE MAGIC OF INCLUSION

Social media is a wonderful platform for this to happen. How many beautiful stories have you seen on social media about people of all-abilities successfully competing in sports, running businesses, working in regular jobs and taking part in all sorts of other community activities.

We need inclusion from everyone so this can continue to be shown and so more people get to live their dreams. So we can all see how great it is when people are given a chance to achieve their goals and be included.

By being inclusive, it gives people and their families the strength and confidence to take steps toward making dreams become reality and to allow their child or the person they care for to participate just like everyone else.

Whether it is sport, work, business or anything else, being kind and showing people it is alright for them to be there are the only things that need to be done. Again, think about how you would feel if people were not being kind to you and how you may react to this.

When we all start seeing more of people's capabilities and just recognising the fact they are people just like everyone else, we begin to understand that everyone is good at something. Anyone can accomplish anything they set their mind to – we all have dreams and aspirations. And I think when we start seeing more of this, inclusion and acceptance will become more of the norm.

We need this to happen so everyone is comfortable doing even day-to-day tasks without feeling like they shouldn't be there or feeling like they shouldn't be having a go.

In my mind, nobody has the right to determine whether or not someone should be somewhere or be doing something. But when people don't behave inclusively, that is exactly what they are doing. They may or may not realise it, but we all need to be more aware of the way we behave towards others and the impact it has on how they feel.

At the end of the day, people, whether they have a disability or not, deserve to feel like they belong. They are, after all, here aren't they? They all have families they belong with and they are all loved as equally as anybody else.

Everyone has something to offer, so make them feel like they deserve to be here and give them a chance.

> ***Benefits of Inclusion:***
>
> *Friendships*
> *Increased social initiations, relationships and networks*
> *Peer role models for academic, social and behaviour skills*
> *Increased achievement of goals*
> *Greater access*
> *Enhanced skill acquisition and generalisation.*
>
> *In fact, social **inclusion** is an **important** 'determinant of health' – without **inclusion**, people are more likely to experience poor health (including poor mental health), loneliness, isolation, and poor self-esteem. ... There are many possible pathways to **inclusion**.*
>
> AskingLot, 'What are the advantages of inclusion?' – *AskingLot*, 5 May 2020.

THE MAGIC OF INCLUSION

I think we need inclusion because it's a chance for people to see how capable everyone actually is and how much fun they can be to be around. Sometimes, people may need some help or slight adjustments may need to be made, but everyone deserves a chance to have a try at something. Once they accomplish it, you don't know where that's going to lead.

An example is with my son Darcy and tenpin bowling. We would take him bowling and he would use the roller to roll the ball toward the pins. We didn't go that often and he was always very happy to use the roller – it never even occurred to me to try and teach him how to bowl without it because I didn't think he would have the strength. More fool me. Once we employed a support worker for Darcy, she started taking him regularly to bowling. Within a couple of weeks, and after being shown how, he was bowling without the roller and getting scores like you wouldn't believe. He gets better and better every time he goes.

Now, if someone didn't include him and show him the steps, we would never have been able to see how much he loves bowling and how capable he is of achieving great results.

It is also very important for families to feel like it's a good idea to put their children out there, to participate in sports, attend social events, and try all types of other activities. If people are not inclusive, it very quickly leads to families not taking their children to events or allowing them to try new things.

This isn't fair.

Everyone deserves to enjoy life and make memories with their loved ones without feeling like they're being a burden on people who don't even really matter.

Let's face it, the people that are not inclusive, are people that aren't in our lives and don't really matter anyway. But they manage to make people feel so uncomfortable that they don't want to take their children anywhere for the fear of that rejection.

I know how it feels … we have been on the receiving end of this and it's not nice. My son also feels this rejection and he doesn't understand it.

Even someone staring, or making a remark is not inclusive. You may be at an event where everyone is included but if someone makes a comment or stares rudely, it makes you feel like you shouldn't be there and therefore, you feel excluded.

Imagine being at an event and having a wonderful time. Then someone makes a negative remark toward you and your child, or even just points and makes a negative gesture. How do you think you would then feel at this event? Immediately the fun has gone, and the day turns into one that you don't remember for the fun, but for the negative behaviour toward you. It's happened to us many times and it is why I try very hard to keep positive because I want our day to remain a good one.

Another example is a story a friend of mine told me once when we were talking about taking our boys out over the holidays. She told me she doesn't take her son out for dinner anymore because of how others make her feel. She said they stare and make comments about him and that makes her feel like they shouldn't be there.

When I asked what her son was doing, she said he was sitting on the floor instead of at the table and people were pointing him out and making awful remarks. One lady, after bending down and talking to her son, then looked at my friend and proceeded to tell her how disgusting her son was. He didn't respond well to whatever she said, and she then made this horrific comment to my friend. This sort of behaviour enrages me.

Why is it their business what he is doing? He wasn't at their table and he wasn't causing a scene by being noisy and disruptive. He was enjoying himself with his family and he wasn't intruding on anybody else's space. He was comfortable and the family were able to enjoy their night out. If they had of tried to make him sit at the table, he wouldn't have responded well. So, by letting him sit on the floor, he was happy and the family were able to enjoy their night. That is, until people started making remarks.

My friend unfortunately has many stories similar to this one and it breaks my heart every time she tells me about them.

These types of comments have a huge ripple effect on everyone around the person too because their loved ones will tell the story of how they were made to feel to friends and family. In turn, it makes people feel like they shouldn't participate for fear of also not being included.

We need inclusion so that everyone can see how easy it is to make someone's day and because everyone deserves to go wherever they want to and experience things as we all do.

Even if they don't achieve success with what they are doing the first time, or if they do things a little differently like sitting on the floor instead of the table, accepting and including them gives them the confidence to keep trying. It is not your business to be making comments about others that don't affect you in any way.

If you are walking past someone, and their child or person they are with is sitting on the floor instead of at the table, give a reassuring look toward them (if you have to look at them at all) or just a casual smile, and it changes the whole situation.

There are some wonderful people out there with fantastic ideas on how to make people feel comfortable in having a go. Sometimes it's only a high five, but it gives someone the happiness and confidence to keep trying.

That is inclusive.

CHAPTER 4

THE INCLUSION SUPERPOWER

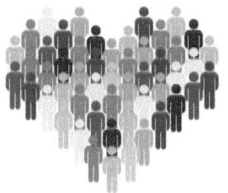

> Coming together is a beginning, keeping together is progress, working together is success.
>
> **HENRY FORD**

From our experience of doing things with our son Darcy, I think EVERYONE benefits from inclusion. In particular, those people that didn't think it would be successful benefit, because it opens their eyes to things they didn't think would be possible.

THE MAGIC OF INCLUSION

When Darcy went on his first camp with the mainstream school he was attending, there was a lot of persuading by me to the school for him to be able to go. Many of the teachers were unsure if he would be okay on camp. They were worried about him not being able to do things and I think therefore they thought he would be a burden on everyone.

Darcy had attended this school part time since Grade Prep and had gone on all of the excursions and taken part in every other activity the kids did at the school.

The teachers were also worried about things like sleeping, behaviours (even though he had been at the school for four years and they knew his personality), participation, missing his family more than the other kids and other things like that.

After many weeks of answering their questions and convincing them of his right to attend, he went on his first camp with them. He was in Grade 3 and was nine years old.

We made a plan that if he didn't cope being away on camp, I would pick him up on the second day and bring him home. This is something that is in place for all kids that attend camp – if they are not coping and want to come home, they can come home.

Originally, they wanted me to take him up and back each day which I flatly refused. I refused this because that would be like going on an excursion and he had been on many of those before successfully. He also would not have understood why the other kids were staying behind while he would have been going home.

I had no doubt about him attending and I knew he would enjoy it just as much as all the other kids. If I didn't think he would cope, I wouldn't have sent him.

I knew he would thoroughly enjoy being with his peers and learning new independent skills, trying new things, socialising on a different level with the other kids. It was an experience I am so happy he got to be part of. He went on four camps with this school from Grade 3 to Grade 6 and they were all extremely successful for him. He had his assistant attend the camps with him, so he had the extra support if he needed it, but she said she mostly just sat back and watched him follow the lead of the other kids and join in like all of them. She was there if he wanted her or needed support, but she said his abilities just shone by following the other children.

I remember the response of the first teacher I saw when they returned from camp as though she was saying it again to me now.

She looked at me with a huge grin on her face and said, 'Wow, what an amazing young man you have there. He was incredible and participated in everything'.

You can imagine how that made me feel. I was so proud and at the same time, felt like saying to them all 'I told you so'.

All the other parents who were also picking their children up had huge smiles on their faces. They could all see that he could do it. He could keep up with the other children and achieve the same goals.

It was truly a wonderful moment and future camps were easier for us to get him to. We faced a few questions of doubt, but we didn't have to convince anyone as much as we did for the first camp. Each year when they returned, a teacher would look at me with pride in their eyes and tell me how amazing Darcy was while they were away.

It's funny because while they were saying how amazing he was, and I was extremely proud, don't get me wrong, I was thinking why is he amazing? Because he did the same things as the other kids that I knew he could do? He's just like all the other kids, learning new experiences and feeling great when they are achieved.

He showed them he could achieve when they didn't think he could. They were amazed because they thought he would need much more support. I was extremely proud and also felt very empowered that our advocating succeeded, and Darcy was able to show them that it was all worth it, and he could do what everyone else was doing, or even just give it a try.

It taught them that it's okay to include and give people a chance. It taught them, it's not going to be a negative outcome, but an amazing learning experience for everyone. Even if Darcy didn't succeed at one of the activities he was trying, it wouldn't have mattered because, he was given a chance to have a go. He may try again and succeed the next time or even the time after that. It doesn't matter. As long as he could try.

When I think back, I remember one of the heads of the school in particular did not want to talk about Darcy going on camp at all. He was quite upset that he was actually going. One time, when I tried to talk to him about it, he put his hand up to my face and said, 'Don't talk to me about it'. I was so upset I almost called the Education Department, but one of the other heads of the school calmed me down.

This particular person was going on the camp with the children and I remember thinking he will probably call me to pick Darcy up just because. Thankfully, this didn't happen. His mind was opened to a whole new world and I was so proud that Darcy made this happen. The following year, this person did everything they could to make Darcy's next camp just as good as the first. It was amazing seeing the transformation.

THE INCLUSION SUPERPOWER

So, I think even when people aren't sure about or open to inclusion, when they see it at its finest, they learn from it and benefit from it.

The person being included definitely benefits from it. You have to remember that inviting someone to the party is not the only thing that needs to happen. If you invite someone to the party, you need to dance with them as well.

> '**Social inclusion** is the process of improving the terms on which individuals and groups take part in society – improving the ability, opportunity, and dignity of those disadvantaged on the basis of their identity.'
>
> The World Bank, 'Social Inclusion',
> The World Bank, no date.
>
> Studies show that **inclusion** is **beneficial** for **all people** – not just for those who get special education services. In fact, research shows that inclusiveness has positive short-term and long-term effects for **everyone**.
>
> The Understood Team, '4 Benefits of Social Inclusion',
> Understood, no date.

So, when someone is included and they have a chance to try something new or just be around friends doing the same thing they are doing, they benefit. It gives them the confidence to keep trying, and when they achieve what they are trying (even if it takes a few attempts), the rewards everyone gets from this is overwhelmingly gratifying.

When Darcy achieves something, he is learning and trying to the best of his ability. He is so happy, and the happiness rubs off on everybody around him.

It also gives him the belief in himself to do it again and even to try other things. Just like all of us when we try something new and we get a good result. It's not different for anyone else if you think about it.

This to me, is the most gratifying thing about inclusion. Seeing the joy on Darcy's face and also the joy for everyone around him. And the confidence it gives him to keep striving to try more things. People who are inclusive definitely get so much out of what they do for others. There are many wonderful organisations that specifically put on events for children who feel like they are left behind.

You have to remember that it's not only children with disabilities that don't always get included. There are many, many children and adults who feel left out and not included.

Life should not be like this.

Just because someone may appear a little different in your eyes, for whatever reason, doesn't mean they really are any different to you or me.

We all have the same feelings. We all have families, we all go to school and/or work and we all have the same emotions – love, happiness, sadness, etc.

So, for someone to exclude someone just because they think they're a little different is crazy to me.

Unfortunately, this happens all the time. But thankfully there are many people advocating for inclusion and the world is slowly getting used to it and becoming better at doing it and understanding its importance.

While social media can be a wonderful platform to show the world what people of all-abilities are capable of, there are still bullies who feel the need to use the private chat messages to make people feel excluded. This is something that we may never be able to stop, however, by providing more inclusive events for people and educating others, it will show them that they are valued and they are in fact good at something. My hope is that by people feeling like this, they will ignore the bullies and not listen to what they say because they will know they are amazing no matter what.

I think if we all do this more often, then hopefully the bullying will begin to be ignored and people can go ahead with their lives.

The media today are definitely on the side of inclusion. Nobody likes to see someone so sad that they don't want to go anywhere or even worse, end their lives.

This sort of thing happens and it's NOT OKAY.

I hope that with further education and letting people know how it makes others feel when they are excluded, we can change the way things are. I know how good it makes people feel when they can see someone achieve something. I see this all the time with my son Darcy.

I take him everywhere. We go to the football, concerts, theatre, movies and he also participates in football, basketball, dance, tenpin bowling and athletics. He learns and improves with his sports all the time and it's wonderful when people see him do something and say, 'Wow look at him go'.

When they say this, I think, 'Yeah, because he plays all the time and he loves what he does. Why shouldn't he be good at things?' I'm proud when they say this about Darcy, but sometimes I wonder why they are surprised.

When we go out, he is extremely well behaved and knows what's expected and I think that's because I've always taken him places so he can experience everything we love to do and the things his brothers have always done. He is my third child, and his brothers were already playing sport when he was born, so he came along too. We would also go to the movies and attend other events regularly, so he was out and about from the moment he joined our family.

For our family, and because my boys had lots of activities they attended in our community, it worked for Darcy. He started coming everywhere with us as soon as he arrived home from the hospital. I do believe, that for us, this is why he is so comfortable going out and being among many people.

I always tried very hard not to let the negativity stop me from taking Darcy out. But I do still get anxious at times depending on where we are going and it's because I'm nervous about the responses we may get. I try to push past these feelings but sometimes it's very difficult and at times I don't take him to certain places. Some people get so anxious, they just can't take their children out and this is what needs to change so they can go out happily and enjoy time with their kids.

I also have tried extremely hard to shelter him from the negativity of others because I don't want him to feel like he shouldn't be somewhere. It seems to have worked because he enjoys everything we do and doesn't seem to worry about others and what they may think.

When he was born, I was running our local Auskick clinic, and his brothers had basketball and football training and many social events. Darcy came to all of them. Everyone accepted him for who he was as a person right from the start.

So, when we experience negative behaviour from people such as stares or bad comments or him not being included in something when we are out, he doesn't understand it. To him, that's not nice … simple. And he's right.

I have tried to change my response to the negative behaviour, to stay positive no matter what, but sometimes I can't. When I do, I feel that everyone leaves the situation on a more positive note. I hope that the people who are negative feel it and go home like that too, and maybe change their outlook and in turn their behaviour.

To me, really everyone benefits from including people. Sometimes we have to show them what to do or explain what is expected, but a lot of the time we don't. That's the beauty of inclusion – letting people have a chance to show you they are just like you.

CHAPTER 5

GROWING STRONG TOGETHER

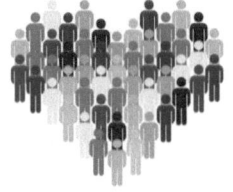

DIVERSITY is having a seat at the table, INCLUSION is having a voice, and BELONGING is having that voice be heard.

LIZ FOSSLIEN

I think there are many, many, many positive results from inclusion and acceptance. I mean, why wouldn't there be?

When you include, it's a positive thing to do. When this happens, everyone can happily go about whatever it is they are doing without having to worry about people leaving them out, making bad comments or even staring and jeering at them.

When people don't include, I think it definitely leaves a bad taste in everyone's mouth.

I mean, a lot of people don't understand why they are not being included. I know Darcy doesn't understand it. He has been involved in so many inclusive things, when he doesn't get included, he doesn't understand why. And now that he is 15 years old, when this happens, it makes him feel awkward and sad. He sticks next to me like glue, and I can feel that he is frightened to come forward.

I don't think anyone should be made to feel this way. It breaks my heart into a thousand pieces.

As I mentioned previously, one of the activities we wanted Darcy to continue to participate in was Auskick. We love our footy in this family and both Darcy's brothers did Auskick and played football. His brother Blake still plays football. Darcy also loves football which is the main reason we wanted him to participate.

Darcy started his Auskick journey at his special school which was run very well and in a safe environment. No judgement.

When this finished being run at his school, we made the decision to take him to our local 'mainstream' Auskick clinic. This clinic always has well over 200 children attending and to say we were nervous about his first day there, would be an understatement.

We went there, not knowing the people who were running it (they are mums and dads volunteering their time). We knew some of the kids in his group because they went to the mainstream school Darcy was attending.

When we arrived, I saw the coordinator straight away and introduced Darcy to her. I was waiting for her to say it may be a bit hard for him because of the size of the clinic and the work the coaches have to do seeing as there are so many kids.

She was the complete opposite. She grabbed the coaches straight away and introduced Darcy to them. She explained he may need a little extra guidance with the skills but apart from that we would be there to help also, and it should all be fine.

It was a breath of fresh air to me. We attended this clinic for five years. Once the first year was over, the kids he participated with went on to junior football. Darcy wasn't up to junior footy at this stage, so continued at the clinic.

So, for the next four years, he had a different group of kids and different coaches and parents. Each year we introduced ourselves and the coaches were more than happy to help Darcy where he needed it.

The inclusion here was amazing. There was nothing too hard and he was treated like all the other kids. The parents always came over and introduced themselves to me and asked me about Darcy. I would tell them how much he loved football and participating with all the other kids. I would also tell them that if their child had any questions, to please ask me. I've always found this a great way for people to learn about Darcy and to understand that, at the end of the day, he wants to learn just like they are learning, and also participate just like them.

The best part of playing with a new group of kids each year was that after a few weeks, one child would always come up and ask us about Darcy. They wanted to know why he needed extra help and why he couldn't kick and pass like they did.

We would explain that he had Down Syndrome which meant it took him a little longer to learn skills. He sometimes would need encouragement from the kids to help him learn.

Each time, from that moment on, Darcy was one of them. They called out to him to pass the ball, they helped him with his skills and even better, they embraced him for who he was.

He wasn't the boy with Down Syndrome. To them, he was Darcy, their footy friend.

By the end of our five years at Auskick, Darcy was kicking and passing the ball just as well as anybody else. The last year, no child asked me questions about him, because to them, he was just Darcy.

We still have kids he attended the clinic with come over when they see us to say hello and see how Darcy is going. They always talk to him and I know that he has friends for life from this experience.

Putting him, and others like him forward like this helps people to understand that everyone is capable, and by giving them a chance, it helps them to shine. They have every right to participate just like anybody else.

So, the end result of Darcy participating in Auskick was that he was included just like everyone else. Nobody ever teased him or mocked him. Instead, they asked questions and then embraced him.

> *The Principles of Inclusion promote equity, access, opportunity and the rights of children and students with disability in education and care and contribute to reducing discrimination against them.*
>
> Inclusive School Communities,
> 'Understanding the Principles of Inclusion', no date

It's very difficult putting your child forward when you think they are going to be judged, teased, or just left out. If you think that is going to happen everywhere you go, you definitely don't want to put them in that situation.

But I think, the more we expose Darcy to things, the more accepting people around him become.

It's not easy just to put yourself out there. It's very difficult at times. You don't want your child being exposed to negative behaviour especially when it's about them and this is what stops a lot of people.

There is no need for people to be judgemental or exclude others from things especially when it doesn't affect them. Most of the time, it doesn't affect them, but they still feel the need to make a comment or a judgement.

Please understand that we are all parents of children.

I think that we all want the same thing – to make memories with our families, to do what we love, and to feel that we can take our children anywhere.

CHAPTER 6

WE MUST DO BETTER

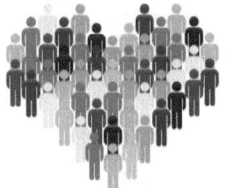

No matter how inclusive we are working towards being, we can always do more. We can always do better.

VICTORIA N. MCGOVERN

I cannot imagine a world where there is no inclusion or acceptance. I am happy that there is inclusion happening even though I know there is so much more room for improvement and education for everyone.

Parents need to be able to do things with their kids without feeling like they are being judged and people need to know it's not alright to judge. As I said earlier, we are all different and if we take the time to realise this, I think including people will happen a lot more freely.

So many people need to be educated on this and thankfully the age we live in now includes tools and platforms that can help so positively with this. With social media for example, we can share wonderful experiences and show the world how capable everyone is.

I shudder to think what it would be like if there were no inclusion or acceptance at all.

I think we would live in a world full of judgement and there would be a lot of people that would not venture outside their homes at all for fear of being ridiculed.

This is one of the major things I love about Darcy's personality and that of his friends ... absolutely NO JUDGEMENT of others. They take everyone for who they are, and not what may be different about them.

If Darcy likes you, you will know immediately because of the caring nature he has and the want to make friends and have fun. If he doesn't like you, for whatever reason (and this doesn't happen often because he takes people how he sees them – no judgement on appearance or ability), you will know this immediately also. He just won't bother with you. He won't pick on you or point and make remarks. He won't do anything. He will go to those he likes and those that like him.

We can't all like each other, but that doesn't mean we have to be judgemental or nasty. I think we should all be more like my son in this regard – if you like someone, let them know and if you don't, just don't bother with them. No pointing or judgemental behaviour – just leave them alone.

WE MUST DO BETTER

When people feel like they're being judged upon because of what they look like or because they may behave a little differently, it makes them avoid going out.

I actually had an experience of this myself in secondary school. I felt as though I was being left out of the group of friends we hung around and I felt as though people were talking about me and pointing at me at times. My solution was that I still went to school, because I had to, but after school, I just stayed home. I didn't even want to go to the milk bar. It was an awful feeling and actually took me a very long time to get over.

Can you imagine your child not wanting to ever go anywhere because they were frightened of what people might say or how they would react about them? Or worse, actually get physically bullied or verbally abused?

It's not a nice feeling to worry about what people might be thinking or going to say just because you have your child out at the movies or at some sort of event, just like everyone else. Or because you want them to participate in sport like all kids love to do.

We all love to do certain things. We all want to create happy memories with our loved ones.

> *'Respecting both similarities and **differences** in others opens doors to many opportunities. You'll learn new things and make better decisions, which in turn will improve your self-confidence.'*
>
> Michael, 'Accepting Other People's Differences', *Ananias Foundation*, 7 January 2019.

Can you imagine what your life and family would feel like if you felt you couldn't participate in things because of how others made you feel? Imagine your child feeling so overwhelmed with negativity from others that they were scared to try something or became that anxious it paralysed them?

Sometimes, it's not always the child that feels this (especially when they are quite young), it's the parent that's taking them out that feels all of this negativity, and the anxiety that comes with this is huge. Feeling like you can't take your child somewhere and saying no to all the invitations that people give you to go with them is a terrible feeling.

I'll bet some of you can't imagine it at all because you may never have experienced it.

You may have been told about it by friends, but you can't really know what it feels like until you've experienced it firsthand. Most of the time I choose to either ignore the judgements or simply smile at people or even sometimes say hello as I have mentioned a few times. It is my way of dealing with the situation and it works every single time for me. The people either smile back and say hello, or they lower their heads and walk away in the opposite direction.

I feel that when I do this, I leave the situation with a clear head and a positive mind. I also feel that when I do this, my son doesn't even recognise that someone was judging him for what they thought he might or might not be able to do, or the way he was behaving.

He is able to go ahead carefree when I remain positive.

Sometimes however, it is very difficult to be like this. We all have down moments and sometimes the exclusion and non-acceptance really grinds at me. I don't understand it, especially when Darcy isn't doing anything that affects those people.

So sometimes I am negative, and I respond negatively.

When this happens, it affects Darcy in that he becomes sad. I also end up leaving the situation in a bad mood, especially if I have said something to the person. And I'm sure they go home not feeling the best, perhaps angry that I have spoken up.

So, I try really hard to focus on being positive. It's taken a long time for me to be like this, but as Darcy has gotten older, he understands and feels negativity. I don't want him feeling this, so I have really focused on being positive for him, and in turn, it's been good for me too.

It's not always easy to do this, depending on the situation that has occurred. An example of where Darcy was affected by the exclusion and my reaction is something that happened in Grade 5 at the mainstream school during the swimming lessons they were doing.

> *They were getting ready for the beginning of Grade 6 where they attend one of our local beaches to do canoeing and other fun and different activities like this.*
>
> *I had filled out my form and paid for the lessons like all the other parents and then came the day of the first lesson. The kids were put in four groups, and they did like a round robin where they tried all the different activities.*
>
> *Darcy's first activity was to go in an inflatable boat in the pool. They were given oars to row around and then had to tip out of the boat and float. They had life vests on and were all very eager to give this a go, including Darcy.*

Now, for some reason, the teacher didn't think Darcy would be capable of this activity and she also had it in her mind he would hit someone with the oar. He has never in his whole life hit anyone with anything. He is not an aggressive child at all, and she had been teaching him PE the whole time he had been at the school.

When she was giving the kids the instructions and handing out the oars, she pointed at Darcy and said, 'You won't have an oar and you won't be going in the boat'.

Now this is a classic example of someone not thinking Darcy would understand their words.

My son looked at her with an extremely hurt and sad look on his face and ran off. He tried to run out of the pool area completely. Darcy is not an absconder and has never run off from me or anyone else. His assistant was furious, and I was also angry but at the same time heartbroken and so very sad that she had made Darcy feel this way.

We took this up with the principal of the school and had a meeting with the teacher. Her excuse was that she didn't know he was going to be participating and she didn't know I wanted him attending the Grade 6 activity the following year. What rot!!!

I told her I had filled in the form and paid my money like everyone else. I told her that I wanted him to participate so he could be ready for the Grade 6 activity and I also told her that I had mentioned it to her previously.

Darcy had participated in every school event during his time at this school, and the swimming activities were no different.

WE MUST DO BETTER

The end result was apologies from her, and Darcy being included in all the activities the following week. My opinion of this teacher changed dramatically after this event and I found it very hard to forgive her for what she had done.

She not only affected Darcy, me and his assistant – she also affected the entire class. The following week when Darcy was in class to participate, one of the kids said, 'Oh, is Darcy joining in this week?'. When I said yes, they all cheered and were so happy he was allowed to join in. I was so happy they were pleased and also the fact they were so vocal about it, because it made this teacher see how these children felt about Darcy.

It also made me a little sad because these children were also upset and hurt about what had happened the week before and I'm sure they didn't understand why it had happened.

We never experienced anything like this again from this teacher, but it was always very tense between me and her after that.

I have always put Darcy forward for things I know he loves to do and things I know he is capable of doing, or even just giving it a red-hot go. I can do this because there is inclusion and acceptance out there. It may not be with everyone, but it is there, and I find if I am putting him forward people seem to look to see what is going to happen at least.

When they see the outcome, I can see the response to inclusion coming out before my eyes.

It's like a light bulb goes off and they can see that it's a good thing to give someone a chance and that Darcy is just like any other child. A young boy wanting to try things and have fun and succeed.

I also have always encouraged people to ask me questions about Darcy and tell their children to ask as well if there's something they want to know. I find that by doing this, people are confident to come forward. One friend told me once she didn't know if it was okay to ask questions. I told her I would much rather people ask and learn than to assume which normally leads to exclusion because they are unsure about what they can offer for Darcy to participate in.

We had great examples of this at the mainstream school with the kids that attended there with Darcy. They were always asking me questions in the first four years. Asking if it was okay to do certain things with Darcy. Asking if they could teach him how to play games and many other things like that.

In the early years at the school, the kids would just let Darcy do whatever he wanted in the games without knowing the rules. They did this just so he could be included. As they got older, they would ask me if Darcy would understand the rules of games they were playing, and if they could try and teach him.

I told them, they may have to repeat themselves for the first few times just to remind him (also because he had played the games for so long without knowing the rules), but he would learn what to do by also watching them.

So, they started teaching him the rules of the games they were playing, and it didn't take Darcy long to learn the rules and play properly with them. They loved that this had happened. His favourite game at the school was four square and once he knew all the rules and played the way they did, all the kids wanted him to play with them. By teaching him, he became extremely good at this game and they loved having him by their side.

If this didn't happen, Darcy would probably have stopped playing as they got older. The kids wouldn't have liked him playing by his own rules. Because of what they did, he was included fully and participated the same way they all did.

If we don't include or accept we are creating a world where children, and their families, don't want to go anywhere. They'll struggle to learn and be scared to even try outside of the safe environment of their school and homes.'

How very sad is that? I would not want my son feeling like this and I'm sure you wouldn't want your child feeling like that either.

CHAPTER 7

SEEING THE GREATNESS

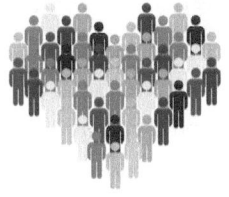

It's not a DISABILITY.
It's a different ABILITY.
ABILITY MINISTRY

Looking at people's abilities and not their disabilities, can make it easier to have inclusion and create an environment that is helpful and diverse.

What I mean is, that when you see their ability first, you are actually allowing yourself to see the person first rather than their disability. You can see what they CAN DO rather than what they CAN'T DO, and can then work on strategies and supports to assist them to learn more and help them to do more. In doing this, you are encouraging them to keep going and feel comfortable in giving things a try.

Everyone has different abilities, and I mean everyone. To focus on what they are capable of at any level is important. It doesn't matter what they can or cannot do, everyone CAN do something.

Allowing a person the chance to participate and achieve, and then celebrating this, makes them want to keep trying new and different things. It gives them confidence. It also gives everyone a chance to see people are not that different to them even if they do need some extra help. They can see they want to do things and learn, just like everybody does.

I know this because I have seen it when Darcy was attending mainstream primary school. We had many wonderful years of inclusion and many lovely stories to share from his time at this school. It's also where I learned to keep trying and to think outside the box a lot more.

We were extremely fortunate to have an assistant that definitely 'thought outside the box' and always had a strategy of how Darcy could join in everything they did even though he couldn't always do it the same way as the other children.

She always came up with a way he could join in and the other kids just ran with it because she always focused on his ability. It was amazing to watch.

Every time this happened, Darcy would try and achieve more than even I expected. Not that I didn't think he could ever do it, but he would end up doing it a lot quicker and trying things he wouldn't have had a chance to if not for the support he received.

Just by changing things up a little when needed, meant that he could always join in. For example, when they would do times tables and each child had to say the next answer (say 7 times table for example), the person in front of Darcy would say the answer 49 and then he would just have to say the number that came next. He would say 50, the class would cheer, and they would continue with their game. He enjoyed sitting in a circle with the kids doing this because he was contributing even though he didn't know his times tables. He was included.

And even though he wasn't doing the times tables, he was participating in math, improving on his counting and having fun with the other kids. The child after him would just continue with the rest of the times table.

One of the simplest forms of inclusion I've seen.

These guys accepted the ability that Darcy had, and included him in the activity. Very simple but very effective. Everyone finished the task happy.

If they focused on his disability and what he couldn't do, the end result would have been very different. It wouldn't have ended as well as when you look at ability. If they decided he couldn't participate in the activity, he would have been sitting on his own watching rather than participating. He would have easily felt bored and left out.

Can you see how simple this activity was to make everyone enjoy it and everyone feel included?

THE MAGIC OF INCLUSION

> *'For so long now we have assumed that physical or mental impairment makes someone **disabled** and based public policy around this assumption, completely ignoring an individual's **ability** in the equation. In an effort to be fair we treated all people with a **disability** equally forgetting that we are as diverse a group as any.'*
>
> Bisset P, 'Change our focus to abilities, not disability, and barriers will fall', *Sydney Morning Herald*, 4 October 2016.

To me, we are all good at some things and not others. And when people can focus on the person and what they can do, they don't worry about what they can't do. They just accept that some people are better at some things than others.

Seeing people's ability is the same thing. Just because people may look or behave a little different, doesn't mean they can't do anything.

They, like everyone else, are better at some things and not others. So, what's the difference?

I'll tell you … there is no difference.

I think we definitely need to focus on the positives which is what people CAN do!!!

Not what they CAN'T do.

It doesn't matter if Darcy can't jump as far as someone else, or run as fast. What matters is that he can do it. So, seeing that he can and accepting how far or fast he can run, is what needs to happen.

SEEING THE GREATNESS

Participating at athletics carnivals at the mainstream school was a prime example of this. Darcy would do every single activity that all the kids were doing. He may have taken a little longer to complete the running, may not have jumped as far in long jump or thrown as far in shot put, but he DID IT! And all the kids cheered him on like they did all of their friends.

It also doesn't matter how he holds a fork, or how he drinks his drink. The fact is that he can still do it.

The list goes on and on … it doesn't matter how he kicks or throws a ball, writes his name, plays with friends, talks or walks. He can still do it. We all walk and talk differently, but nobody ever makes a big deal about it.

I am left-handed and hold my pen differently to a lot of other people, especially those who are right-handed. When people see me write, they comment that I hold the pen weird and ask me if it's uncomfortable. It used to annoy me because I wondered why they needed to comment, but now I just show them how neat my writing is. It takes the focus away from what they have just said to me and they concentrate on my end result. It doesn't matter how I do it.

When someone has a disability, those that are non-inclusive, think it's okay to be judgemental about these things. It's not okay. They're not hurting anyone in the way they do things, they're not causing you any problems, so just leave them be if you can't be positive.

If you can't focus on what they can do and support this, then my advice is just to leave them alone.

Seeing ability rather than disability (as inclusion and acceptance) makes the person strive to keep going and not have to worry about what people are thinking. When people feel like they can keep going about what they are doing, and keep trying, they will always get better at what they are doing anyway. It's like the old saying, 'practice makes perfect'.

My son Darcy has Down Syndrome, but this does not in any way define him. It is just a part of him. He may not be able to do things like everyone else or how people think he should, but I tell you he gives most things a red-hot go. And if he doesn't succeed the first time, we definitely don't give up.

Being like this with him, seeing his ability, has allowed him to have the confidence to try lots of different things. I know his ability and I put him forward for things I know he will have a go at. Doing this has given him the confidence to try other things as well.

When people see what he has achieved, whether it be in person or on social media, I think this helps them to see that anyone can do anything. So, cheer people on no matter how good or bad they are at things. At least they're having a go and trying things.

If you see the ability and not the disability, it also opens your eyes to a lot as well – it shows you what remarkable things anyone can achieve.

So, this comes to acceptance and inclusion again. Doing these two things helps you to see people's abilities and not their disabilities.

I don't know where we would be with Darcy (and I'm sure my friends with children with disabilities would be the same) if people weren't accepting and inclusive. He wouldn't have the chance to try things and learn, and he wouldn't have the chance to show people how able he is. Just like everyone else.

SEEING THE GREATNESS

So, open your eyes and hearts and step into our world for a while. Open yourself to see the person and not their disability. I guarantee you will not only be surprised, but it will definitely make you understand how important it is and it will definitely make you feel happy for them.

CHAPTER 8

A PLACE TO SHINE

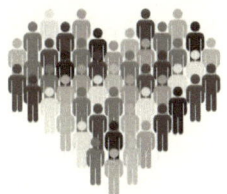

How does a sensory room help? A sensory room can provide a low stress, fun environment for an individual to work through their emotions and reactions to certain stimuli.

AUTHOR UNKNOWN

Part of being accepting and inclusive is also allowing spaces for people to go if they feel like they are becoming overwhelmed with where they are, such as crowded places, or somewhere with loud noise or bright lights. Somewhere they can go that is quiet and they can unwind a little, catch their breath and regroup before they go back to where they were.

This doesn't only happen to people with seen disabilities. People living with autism, high levels of anxiety or other mental health issues can feel overwhelmed in some circumstances.

In fact, we all need a break sometimes, like when we are at a party and just need five minutes of quiet before we rejoin the group. People can become overwhelmed when they are in very busy places where there is a lot of activity, with people buzzing around and noise.

I have seen this in people with seen disabilities and disabilities you cannot see. When you can see a disability, some people are more patient and understanding because they have a visual. If a disability cannot be seen, this is where judgement comes in, especially if they have a meltdown.

This is why a sensory area for people to go to is so important.

Thankfully, many places are now including sensory areas for children and adults to go to just to sit and gather their thoughts and desensitise before they re-enter the event. Just to sit on your own sometimes without lots of things happening around you and have some calming distractions, can turn a situation from bad to good very quickly.

In children, sometimes when they get overwhelmed, they have what is called a meltdown.

Again, if there is a visible disability, many people accept what is happening to the child and will go about their business if they don't offer help.

If there is an unseen disability, people immediately become judgemental and make snide remarks or give horrible glares.

This then puts the parent in a very uncomfortable frame of mind (as if they weren't already in one) and causes them more anxiety than what they're already experiencing.

This is why sensory areas are so important. It is somewhere we can take our children quickly and safely. The child usually feels calmness pretty quickly because they can see they are now in a safe environment. The parent can then gather their thoughts and work towards taking their child back into the event where they can all enjoy things most of us take for granted.

The AFL have developed sensory areas which is wonderful because many of us, particularly in Victoria, have grown up going to the football and want our children to experience the fun of going to a game live rather than just watching on TV.

Larger family shows, like the Melbourne Show, are also starting to develop sensory areas. Again, it allows us to take our children to things we grew up going to. They don't have to go on rides or anything like that, but just to go to something like this and experience all the wonderful fun things going on is enough.

A friend and I attended a small carnival once with Darcy and her daughter. It was unplanned but it was a small carnival and didn't look too busy. I thought it would be a great experience for us together.

Darcy is a child that has started to enjoy going on rides, so at this event, he went on rides and had a great time. His friend isn't as confident going on rides, but she had just as much fun playing the arcade games and interacting with some of the people at the carnival.

I remember her mum being nervous about going to this carnival because she knew her daughter wouldn't go on the rides and she worried about what people would think. It was the complete opposite. People could see she enjoyed the games and music that was playing, and they all made a point of talking to her and making her feel included at the event.

So, it doesn't matter what people can or can't do. Just to be able to go to an event and know there is a safe place if they get overwhelmed is the best thing for them and their families.

> *'Time in a sensory room helps children improve their visual, auditory and tactile processing, as well as fine and gross motor skills. By providing a sense of calm and comfort, sensory rooms help children learn to **self**-regulate their behaviours, which ultimately improves focus.'*
>
> American School for the Deaf, 'The Benefits of Sensory Rooms for Children With Autism and Social/Emotional Challenges', *ASD*, 21 May 2019.

It isn't a bad thing that people need to take time out to adjust their thoughts. I think it is a good thing. It allows them to also identify when they do become unsettled or overwhelmed. It helps them identify their feelings and react in an appropriate way to help calm themselves.

Many people don't know what a sensory area is. It is not just a room with a few chairs in it, or an empty room. It is a wonderful space filled with colours, quiet games, bean bags to chill out on, relaxing music and lights. Somewhere a person can feel calm as soon as they enter and see all the lovely colours and hear the nice calming music. Games can quickly distract children from the negative feelings they have and help them concentrate on something else.

The music and colours can relax immediately. Even stress toys, colouring books and pencils and other things like this can be put into a sensory room. Something they can grab hold of straight away and sit with.

An empty bare room, to me, wouldn't help to relax someone. If I walked into an empty room feeling anxious, I would immediately start to feel more anxiety. Where do I sit, what do I do? Why is it empty?

And if there are other people in there, they would all be doing the same thing. Standing there looking around wondering what to do next.

When you enter a room with appealing sights, sounds and activities and see a few others there already desensitising, you relax and find something to do or somewhere to just sit comfortably.

With all of the calming lights, music and comfortable surroundings, someone can walk into one of these rooms and immediately identify with something they like that will calm them. This allows them to take their mind off what was making them feel anxious.

If you are a parent taking a child into an area like this, you can also scan the room straight away and find an area you know your child will be comfortable in. Take action and start the calming process so you can all go on and enjoy the rest of your day.

Some people wouldn't think about something like a sensory area and may not know what they are. They are not just for children or people with disabilities – they are for anyone who feels a bit overwhelmed in the space they are in.

There is no discrimination here in a sensory area. Everyone is welcome.

They definitely are a very calming area as soon as you enter them. There is something in them for all the senses to begin to relax and unwind.

Many of my friends ask the event organisers before they attend whether they have a sensory area. It makes a huge difference to them and can determine whether or not they will attend the event. I'm not just talking a handful of people, I'm talking many, many people.

These are potential sales at the gate that the organisers are missing out on.

Many organisers don't even realise about sensory areas until they are asked the question. A friend asked an event whether they had a sensory area and was told they had an empty room for people to go into if they needed to. My friend explained to them that this was not a sensory area, and she is now working with them on future events to ensure the space they provide is suitable for everyone who needs to access it. This is amazing as now many more people can attend their event without worrying what they will do if their child begins to not cope with their surroundings.

So, even if you don't need a sensory area, maybe ask the organiser if they have one to get the ball rolling if they don't.

Even most parks are not safe for some families and their children. Not because of sensory areas, but because of a lack of fencing around the playground. Especially if the park is near a busy road or has a body of water nearby.

You wouldn't normally think of something like this until you enter the world of disability. A lot of my friends have children that will run and keep running. If there are fences available at parks, their child can run without their parent worrying about losing them, or even worse, running onto a busy road. Their child can also enjoy the area without their parent having to constantly be at them to tell them where they can or cannot go, therefore making them relaxed to enjoy the space they are in.

How sad is it that some families don't take their kids to a park because they don't feel safe? Their children are missing out on what every child should be able to experience.

Work is happening and slowly more and more councils are providing fenced areas at their parks for these families.

How wonderful is that?!

Such a simple thing but something that makes such a HUGE difference in people's lives. Much like the sensory areas.

It's not only children with disabilities and their families that benefit from this, but all families. Many children, whether they have a disability or not, run off from their families and can't be found. If there is a fenced playground you can go to, at least you know they won't go too far away before you can find them.

I know lots of families that would go to these parks that are fenced above the ones that are not. My friend is also working with councils trying to improve this area as well. It is a slow process to see changes, although it shouldn't be. However, she is being listened to and there has been some action happening.

More and more, people are encouraging families to take their children with disabilities out, but they aren't willing to make a few changes here and there to make it safe for them to do so.

Back to sensory areas … even the supermarkets are recognising the need to provide a safe environment for people to shop without feeling overwhelmed.

Sensory hours have been introduced at supermarkets where the lights are dimmed, and the sounds are lowered. I've shopped during one of these times and it actually makes it a lot more relaxing to do your shopping.

Again, thinking outside the box is something that people are starting to do so that all families can go and enjoy the things most of us take for granted.

CHAPTER 9

GETTING THERE, DOING THAT!

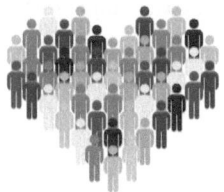

I believe in accessibility. I believe in honesty and a culture that supports that. And you can't have that if you're not open to receiving feedback.
MINDY GRASSMAN

Accessibility is a huge part of inclusion and acceptance because if people can't access where they are going, then they can't be a part of it. Many places think they are providing accessible areas, however, they are not fine-tuning it.

This is often true of parking at shopping centres and other venues. I have seen many accessible parking bays where I wonder how they are 100% accessible for people.

All public places must provide these for people to be able to access the venue whether it be a supermarket, shopping centre, restaurant or wherever they may be going.

We can see the accessible parking bays are there however, not all of them meet the fully accessible criteria.

I have seen many that are not close to the entrance as well as parking spaces that are close to the door but have obstructions around them. The accessible parking areas are meant to be in a space that allows enough room for people to exit their vehicle and gain easy access to where they are going.

A friend recently shared a photo of an accessible parking bay where there was an obstruction that would cause the person not to be able to get out of their car easily and then they would have to walk back onto the road and around the obstruction to then gain entry into the venue.

It's plain to see the quotas for accessible parking bays are being met but they do need to really think about the best way to make them fully accessible and not just place them in areas without planning it properly.

GETTING THERE, DOING THAT!

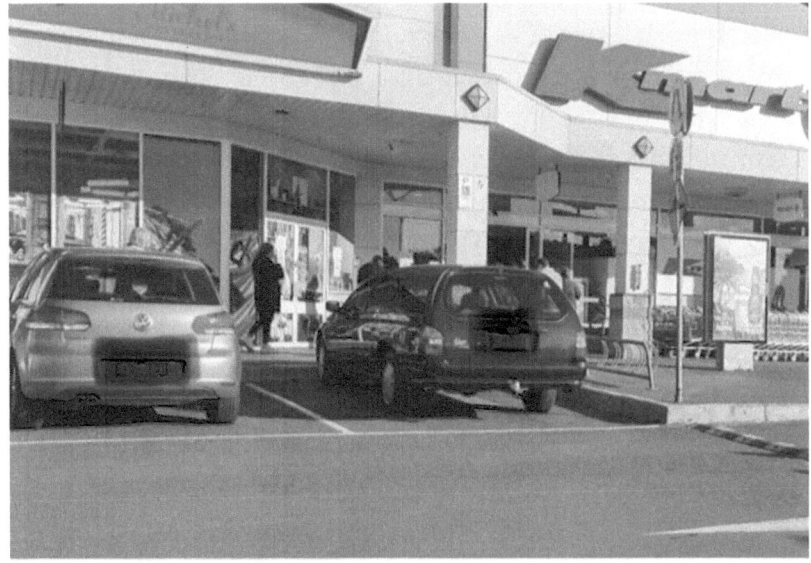

With access to venues, a good example is from a friend of mine who lives in a wheelchair. She always rings ahead to make sure there are accessible toilets for her to use and to also ensure she is able to get into the venue.

One time she was going out with friends and contacted the venue to ensure she would be able to go with her friends and enjoy a night out. They assured her she would have access to all areas of the venue and that there was a disability toilet for her to access.

When she got to the venue, she was able to enter the premises with her friends and find a suitable table. They were all having a great night until she needed to go to the bathroom. When she got to where they had the toilet, she could see there was one there, but she could not get into it with her wheelchair. Therefore, the area was not accessible for her.

The venue had supplied the disability toilet for patrons however, they had not considered all of the types of wheelchairs that would need to access it. She was not happy and told the venue that they were not fully accessible for everyone.

There are many different examples of where people may struggle to enter a venue or a shop because it hasn't been laid out well to be able to include everyone.

An example with Darcy that I can share is also about the toilet areas within shopping centres and other venues. Darcy was incontinent until recently so I would need to access the disability toilets to change him when we were out.

This was fine when he was small because I would be able to use the change table area supplied. I didn't even consider myself what was going to happen when he became older.

And, as you guessed it, as he grew and became older, I was not able to use the change table area that is always attached to a wall and folds down. He was too long, too heavy and too wide for the area.

The only thing I was able to do was to lay him on the concrete floor to change him. This was a nightmare. He didn't like it, he felt unsafe and it was hard, cold and dirty.

After the first time, to make sure I would be able to change him, I used to take a blanket or some towels with me so I could lay him on the floor. Many of my friends have had the same problem with the change facilities and it is actually really demeaning for them and their children.

I think the solution to this problem is that perhaps a sturdier and larger change area be developed and installed in the toilets at these venues. Perhaps a fold out portion in the wall that is larger in size

GETTING THERE, DOING THAT!

and sturdy enough to take extra weight. This way, you don't have to use the floor to change your child or whoever it is you are caring for.

It is also extremely important to ensure the accessible toilet areas are clear from obstructions and well maintained so they can be used at all times. If there are obstructions or the area cannot be used, what do you think happens? The person who is trying to access these areas cannot and has to try and gain access to the other toilet areas which are near impossible to gain entry into. This is why there are accessible toilets.

Unfortunately, some shopping centres and other venues seem to continually have trouble keeping these areas fully accessible and it needs to change. It's very difficult and people shouldn't have to struggle just to use the bathroom.

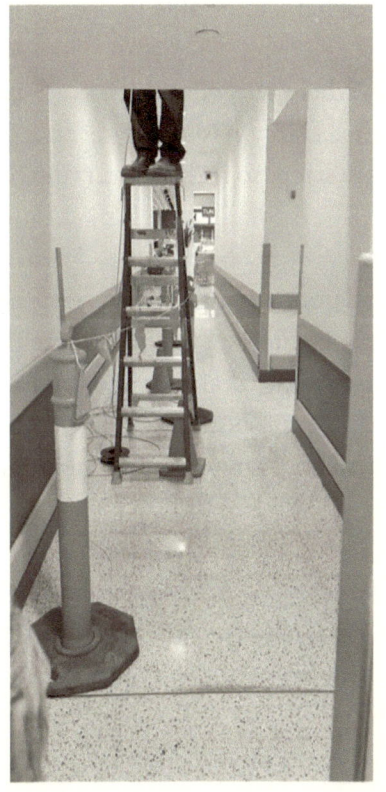
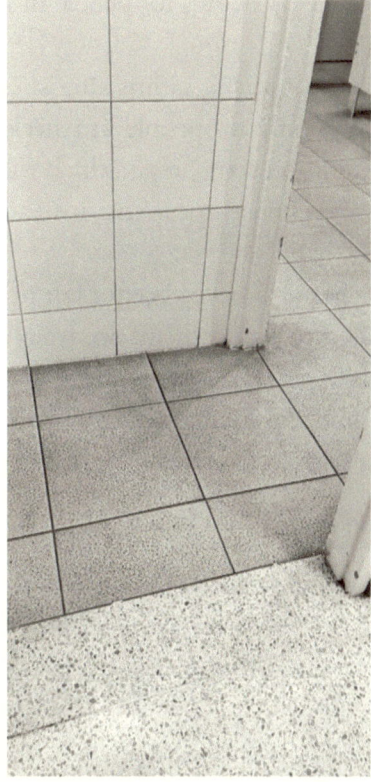

THE MAGIC OF INCLUSION

We have to be aware of accessibility everywhere we go, both at outdoor places and indoor places. It isn't easy for everyone to get to certain areas, and it is important for people to be able to access everything so they can enjoy days out with friends and family.

Beaches have always been difficult however, there are specialised bikes that will allow people to go onto the beach. These are expensive however, and not everyone is able to purchase one. There are now a lot of beaches that are installing specialised ramps for people in wheelchairs to access. I love this and it's wonderful to see my friends now being able to enjoy a day out at the beach.

Many parks are including more and more paths, so accessibility is there for many more than there was before, as well as councils installing the specialised swings for people in wheelchairs to be able to use.

It is great seeing ramps almost everywhere we go, and these are not always only for people in wheelchairs. Darcy has always been a bit nervous on stairs, especially if they are steep, so if there is a ramp, we always choose to use that instead.

He has also never been a fan of escalators and has always been too scared to go on them. So, we always need to be aware of where the lifts are. Sometimes they are not close to the escalators and are hard to find. So better signage would help here especially when you are out with friends and have to meet them on the floor you are going to.

> '***Accessibility*** *can be viewed as the 'ability to access' and benefit from some system or entity. ... This **is** about making things **accessible** to all people (whether they have a disability or not).'*
>
> My Blind Spot, 'Accessibility Defined', *MBS*, no date.

Most supermarkets have now improved accessibility by making their aisles and point of purchase wider and accessible for everyone. There is nothing worse than going somewhere, even with a pram, and not being able to move around the store properly.

It's made life easier for many people.

Cafes and restaurants must also make sure there are areas where everyone can gain access easily. Going for a coffee or a meal and being able to go straight to an area where you are comfortable is so important. It definitely makes going out a lot more enjoyable for all patrons.

Being able to get around the venue to order meals, drinks and to access the bathrooms is something that needs to also be considered. People must be able to access all areas when out.

Imagine going out for dinner with family and friends, being able to enter the venue and be seated comfortably and then not being able to access the area to purchase meals and drinks. People would then need someone else to do it for them which is not ideal especially when they are strong and independent people or if someone is teaching their child independent skills by ordering for themselves. Having to rely on others isn't something everyone wants or needs to do unless it is absolutely necessary.

Transport is another area that has become more accessible for people with taxis, buses and trains however, it was not always like this and there are still many improvements needing to be made here. I'm pleased there is progress, but much more needs to be done.

I was told recently by a friend about her friend that is blind and has a guide dog to assist her wherever she goes. She ordered an Uber and the driver refused her entry into his car because of her dog. I couldn't believe my ears because firstly, I didn't think this could happen because her dog is an extension of her to assist her when going out. And secondly, I couldn't believe the rudeness of this. Imagine how this made her feel. Enraged I would imagine. How did she get to where she needed to go?

This sort of thing shouldn't happen. People should be able to access any type of transport to be able to get to where they want to go.

It is important when planning an outing with someone to know that you will be able to get there safely and without any issues or problems. It's also important to know that where you are going is a safe place where you can access all areas.

Even with Darcy, until recently, we have had to be mindful of taking him to certain places because he was not sure or felt unsafe. It is much better now for him because most places accommodate everyone, and nothing is too hard when we ask for assistance.

There are still some barriers we encounter but it is good to see things improving.

Keep in mind too, if accessibility is an issue for someone when you are out and you approach management or staff, it is important to be kind and try and resolve the issue. I have found from experience and from watching my friends, that there is always a solution to most problems. You just have to listen and think outside the box.

CHAPTER 10

TOGETHER WE STAND

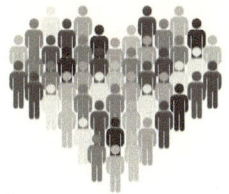

Strength lies in differences, not in similarities.
STEPHEN R COVEY

I may be repeating myself a little, but the message I want to get across is so important.

I feel the need to explain inclusion and acceptance is so vital. Sharing how it makes people feel when they are accepted and included, and the wonderful things that can happen when it occurs, I think helps people to broaden their thoughts and perspective around the experiences of others.

We don't all cross paths with people with disabilities, so we don't all get to see how much like everyone else they really are. Their feelings, thoughts, actions and everything else, are the same as those we all feel and go through.

Outcomes from including people come in many shapes and forms …

Lessons

Pride

Happiness

Achievement

Acceptance

Just a small selection of outcomes, but they have something important in common – they are all positive. These are all things that make everyone feel proud and happy about what they're doing. Both the people providing the inclusive activity and the people that are being included.

And what about the outcomes if we don't include …

Sadness

Feeling alone

Anger

Worthlessness

Hurt

All negative feelings where everyone walks away not feeling good at all.

I know which I prefer.

> *'Some of the benefits of inclusion for children with (or without) disabilities are friendship skills, peer models, problem-solving skills, positive self-image, and respect for others. This can trickle down to their families as well, teaching parents and families to be more accepting of differences.'*
>
> Aguliar E, 'The Benefits of Inclusion', *Easterseals*, no date.

I prefer to see my son enjoying the same things everyone else gets to enjoy and having the options available to try new things. I love to see him, and anyone for that matter, achieving things and feeling proud of what they've done.

I also love seeing the reactions from others when someone they didn't think would be able to do something, actually did it and did it well.

And even aside from including people with disabilities, it goes for everyone.

> You have to stick up for what you believe in. And that, to me, is the biggest thing you can do about driving inclusion.
> **GINNI ROMETTY**

There are many kids and even adults that feel like they're alone and don't have any friends or anyone to enjoy things with.

I don't like seeing this at all because I don't this it's fair. And I don't think anyone would like to see someone they love go through this.

Sometimes I think you have to ask yourself how you would feel if this were happening to someone you knew or someone in your family that you loved.

And also ask yourself, why is it a problem to just include someone? You don't have to be their best friend. Sometimes just saying hi and smiling at someone rather than pointing and staring is all you have to do.

Very simple isn't it?

CHAPTER 11

SPEAK NO EVIL

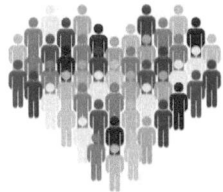

In a world where you can be anything,
BE KIND.

CELEBRATE T21

Be mindful of what you are saying to a parent of a child with additional needs. Remember, it is their child you are talking about.

Have you ever thought about what it would feel like if someone were to say something derogatory to you about your child that they wouldn't say to someone else? This is a huge factor when it comes to inclusion and something that happens a lot in the world of disability.

Something like, 'I'm sorry'.

Has anyone ever said that to you when you have told them you are expecting a baby or when you have told them about the baby you have just brought into the world?

When I was pregnant with Darcy, there was a possibility Down Syndrome may be diagnosed. We decided we wanted to find out before his birth because we wanted to tell our family and friends and we wanted to start learning and getting ready for anything he may need when he arrived. We also wanted happiness when he entered the world, not sadness, worry and doubt.

We got the diagnosis at 15 weeks and we began telling people immediately.

I actually wish I had of started charging for every time someone said, 'I'm sorry'. I would be rich.

I totally understand that people don't mean anything negative by this comment. It is something we all say when we hear sad news or if we don't know what else to say. I don't get angry about people saying it, but I do want people to stop and think before they say this next time they are told a friend has a child with a disability. It happens very often and has happened to all of my friends.

I want people to think about what they would normally say to someone who is expecting or who has just had a child. Take the disability out of it.

So, instead of saying, 'I'm sorry', say 'Congratulations'. That is what we want to hear.

We are bringing, or have brought, our child into the world and we want congratulations. We love them just like anyone loves their child.

Unfortunately, some of this negative language comes from medical professionals, although, in these current times, I am seeing more and more positive language coming here. The medical professionals are the first point of call and if they start the journey on a negative tone, it seems to set the course for a while. If they change the way they deliver their language, the course changes to a more positive one.

When I was pregnant with Darcy and we received the diagnosis, both of the medical professionals I was seeing also said, 'I'm sorry'. I told them they shouldn't be sorry, and everything would be alright. Can you imagine that? Me telling them that everything will be alright. They should have been reassuring me.

As medical professionals, they have an obligation to tell you your options regarding the pregnancy when you receive a diagnosis like Down Syndrome.

When I was pregnant with Darcy, I remember telling them I understood they needed to tell me and I sat and listened. I didn't really take a lot of notice because we were never going down the road of termination. I remember walking away from those appointments (because there were two doctors I was seeing), feeling very flat and sad. I was sad for them because they had to tell people this and I was sad because of what they told me that the steps for this were.

I wasn't ready for the next few appointments where they kept telling me about termination. I had already told them we had discussed it and we were not terminating. We had also started planning the things Darcy would need when he was born and had been going to a support group where we met many families and their children, and we are still friends today (much like a first mums' group).

Doctors need to take the negativity out of their language and talk to people in a more positive tone, like they would if the child were a typical child.

Instead of saying, 'I'm sorry, I have bad news' perhaps say something like, 'Something has shown up in your results I would like to talk to you about'. Then proceed to tell them the diagnosis and talk to them about the supports that are available rather than go straight into the option of termination.

I think if the initial language used is positive, it changes how everything progresses for the parent. They begin their journey on a positive note with resources instead of being surrounded by negativity and feeling like what they are about to enter into is not right.

The world of disability for us has been amazing. The people we have met, and continue to meet, are very supportive, non judgemental and extremely caring of everyone's needs and what they are going through. I am extremely grateful for all the wonderful people we have met and keep meeting.

The other part of language we need to consider is when we are talking directly to the person with the disability.

We have to remember that they are a person living with whatever condition they have been diagnosed with. They are not the disability.

> *'Put the person first, and the impairment second (when it's relevant). Other phrases that are growing in popularity and acceptance are: "person living with disability".'*
>
> Australian Network of Disability, 'Inclusive Language', AND, no date.

Also remember that just because someone has a disability and additional needs, doesn't mean they don't understand what you are saying. They may not respond the way some of us would, but believe me, they definitely understand.

Imagine if someone were to refer to your child as 'it' right in front of them. How would that make you feel? And more importantly, how it would make your child feel?

Being spoken about as though they are an object rather than a person is one of the most degrading things someone can do to another person.

I asked some of my friends with children with Down Syndrome if they would share with me some of the remarks they had encountered with regards to their child. I share some of them below, with my reflections on these comments:-

'He doesn't look typically downs.' I don't know what this comment means. What is typically downs? Don't we all look different? Like, do people say, 'He doesn't look like a typical boy'? That's the sort of thing that comes to mind when I hear a comment like this.

'He's always going to be a baby.' I've met a lot of young children, teenagers and adults with Down Syndrome and they are NOT babies *and don't behave like babies. They attend school, play sports, have jobs or are learning job skills. I don't think babies do this do they?*

'How severe is it?' This comment is made from lack of knowledge about Down Syndrome. There are three types of Down Syndrome – Trisomy 21 (the most common), Mosaic and Translocation. They are all the same chromosomal syndrome with the cells attaching differently in each one, and people that live with Down Syndrome are like everyone else – they learn differently.

The classic, 'I'm sorry'. I spoke about this at the beginning of this chapter. I honestly think people say this because they don't know what else to say. I would have liked to have heard 'Congratulations' when they heard about my son. I'm sure my friends would have liked the same. Or even just ask things about the child, like how old is he, is he a good baby, does he sleep through the night. Questions you would ask any other mother about her child.

'He's always so happy.' This comment is definitely due to a lack of knowledge and people think this because when they see someone with Down Syndrome out and about, it's usually when they are doing something they enjoy. My son, for instance, is not always happy. He has all the same emotions as anybody else and he shows them like anybody else would. I would say my son is very loving, caring and empathetic, but definitely not always happy. He gets upset and angry too.

'He's so special.' I think every person is special in their own way. With my son, he has an amazing sense of how people are feeling and responds in a very caring way. I think this happens because he looks at people and things without any blockers. His feelings are pure, what you see is what you get. So, I guess if that's special, then yes, I guess he and his friends are special. But I think we all hold very special qualities in different ways.

'He's very good looking for one of those.' This was a comment made by a locum paediatric consultant on first meeting a young man with Down Syndrome. WHAT?!!! I know that if I was this young man's mother, I would have immediately said he is a person or what is one of those? I don't understand how anyone, let alone a medical practitioner, could say something like this.

'We've got one of those on our camp, the kids play with it.' This is a comment made by a gypsy selling lavender as she pointed to my friend's son. WOW! Do people even realise they are speaking about a human being with feelings? Do they realise they are speaking to a mother about her son? Would they like their child being referred to as 'it'? I wouldn't have been able to contain myself if this had of been said about my son. I don't know how my friend responded to this, but I'm guessing it wouldn't have been pretty.

'He doesn't look Downs.' I have had this comment made about my son too. For many years I didn't know how to respond and then I came up with 'No, he looks like his brothers'. That turned the comment back on the person who made the comment, and they then didn't know what to say. I don't think this comment is a nasty comment. Again, I think it is a comment made when someone doesn't know what else to say.

'Sorry, but he's never going to get a proper job, he has Down Syndrome.' The boy this comment was made about is now a successful model, he is a coach in rugby and soccer, and he is a trainee baker. Many people with Down Syndrome and other disabilities run successful businesses and have great jobs. Oh, this comment was made by a doctor. Blows my mind.

'She's always going to have health issues, it's never going away.' Ummmm? There are many people who have medical issues without

having Down Syndrome. I know a lot of people whose children don't have Down Syndrome but do have medical issues they have been tackling for many years. And most medical issues can be treated well, and people live great lives with them.

'Oh look, a real life retard.' This comment was made by a 17-year-old toward a 4-year-old. Why? This was not said to my son and I don't know how my friend responded, but I think I would have punched him in the face. A comment like this fuels anger and most people I know would respond very quickly and without thinking, defending their child. I seriously cannot believe this was said to someone's child.

'There's no excuse for a child like this to be born in this day and age.' This was a comment made by a medical professional to a mother. I have also had this said to me. My son brings so much to our family and community and he is a valued member of both. He does things like other children, so I don't know why he shouldn't be here. I could probably write a small book about this comment. It actually enrages me.

A friend's mum said to her, 'We've got one of them in the family too'. My friend said the moment was very awkward, but they knew she didn't mean anything nasty by the comment. I don't know what 'one of them' is because last time I looked, everyone that I know that lives with Down Syndrome is a person.

A good friend of mine had this comment made to her – 'Did you actually give birth to him? Did you have testing done beforehand?' My friend was in shock that someone would actually say something like this. What sort of questions are they? It dumbfounded me when she told me. I believe this woman also said to my friend, 'How could someone so beautiful have a baby like that'. I think it's very sad this woman felt this way about my friend's gorgeous boy.

These comments are just a few of what my friends and I have heard from others with regard to our children. I honestly think I could write an entire book just with things people have said.

I truly hope people don't realise what they are saying is so hurtful and mean. I really hope they are saying these things out of lack of knowledge.

Unfortunately, this is not the case for many of these comments.

I always say, remember, these children you are making comments about are OUR CHILDREN. We love them just as much as you love your children, and they mean the world to us. They are very important members of our families.

So, please think before you speak or make comments.

Some people are not confident enough to say something back whereas others will give you a mouthful you probably aren't expecting.

Be mindful of what you say and also remember, everyone is a person first, just like you and me.

Everyone has feelings and no-one likes having them hurt. Just think about what you are going to say before you say it. Sometimes, people just don't think through what they are about to say to a parent about their child.

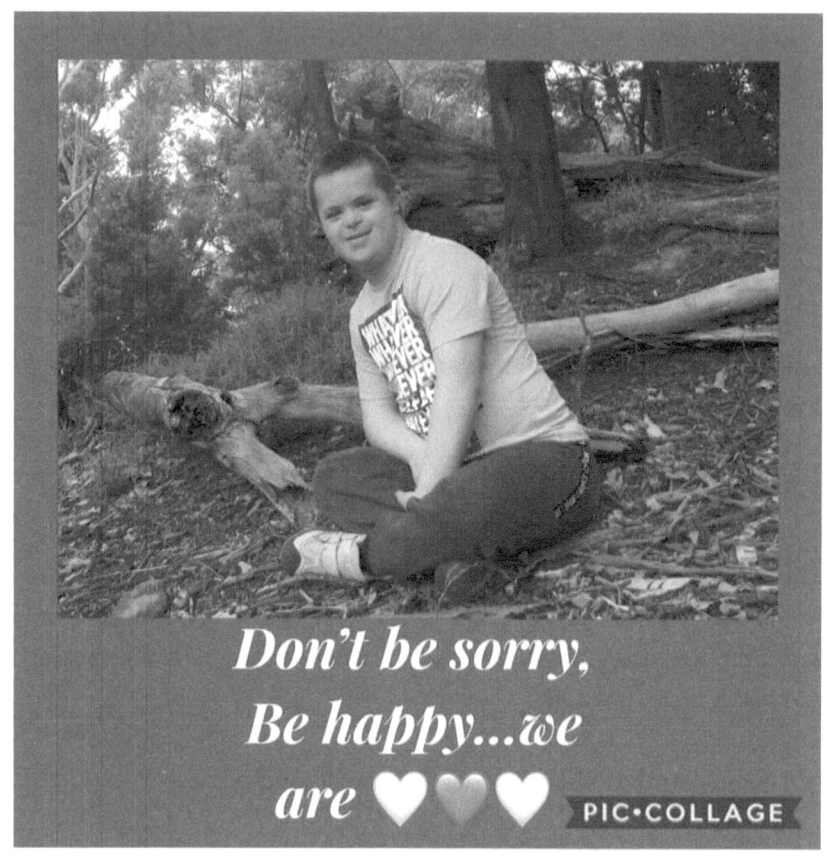

CHAPTER 12

WE CAN, SO WE MUST!

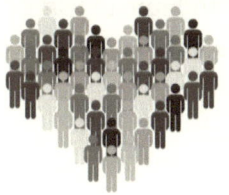

Advocacy: to change 'what is' into 'what should be'.
AUTHOR UNKNOWN

It is very common for people with disabilities to have an advocate assist them to stand up for their rights and speak on their behalf when they cannot.

Advocacy is speaking up for people individually or as a group when they cannot speak up for themselves. It is a process of empowering people by supporting and representing them towards independence and protecting their rights.

Advocates do not take over a person's life; they simply act on their behalf to make sure their rights are being upheld and they are not being discriminated against. Advocates can also work with people with regard to their goals in life and helping them set in place a step-by-step approach to achieve those goals.

People with disabilities are one of the more likely groups of people who require an advocate to assist them when it comes to speaking up for their rights, especially when something has happened at school, in the workplace or even with family and friends.

According to the Australian Human Rights Commission Convention on the Rights of Persons with Disabilities, every person has the right to:

- Freedom of speech
- Choice of living
- Being free from abuse or neglect
- Freedom of culture, religion and language
- Protection from the law

People also have the right to:

- Personal choice and independence
- The ability to care for themselves
- Contribute to all decisions that affect their lives
- Access to the community and the facilities and services in that community
- Choice of needs.

There are different types of advocacy available to suit a range of needs including:

Self-Advocacy where you can speak up for yourself. You can also use an advocacy service to help you understand your rights and how to go about speaking up for yourself. They can be with you when you are dealing with the situation but allow you to speak for yourself.

Individual Advocacy where an advocate will work together with someone to sort out any big problems they may have experienced. These sorts of situations can happen anywhere – at school, work, in the community and even in the home.

Citizen Advocacy is where a member of the community will voluntarily assist a person with a disability to represent their interests and help them obtain a good outcome.

Group Advocacy is usually provided by an organisation who represents a group working towards getting rights and entitlements for people.

Legal Advocacy is where your rights are assisted by a legal representative. This usually happens when something cannot be resolved and ends up being taken to court to get a resolution.

There is also **Community Advocacy** where someone will work on behalf of their community to make areas more accessible and inclusive. An example of this is getting fences around community parks as I mentioned earlier. There are many children (not only with disabilities) that will run off from their parent or carer. Getting suitable fencing around the park area ensures the children are safe and their families can enjoy a trip to the park like everyone else.

Advocacy seeks to ensure that all people in society are able to:

- *Have their voice heard on issues that are important to them.*
- *Protect and promote their rights.*
- *Have their views and wishes genuinely considered when decisions are being made about their lives.*

Advocacy Focus, 'What is Advocacy?', *Advocacy Focus*, no date.

Some people with disabilities require an advocate to assist them because they may need help with communication. An advocate will assist the person to voice their concerns and relay this to the other party involved.

There are also times where someone may not feel confident in standing up for themselves depending on what has occurred. If it is a workplace incident, they may be fearful of losing their jobs. It is the advocate's role to make sure the person knows they are entitled to stand up for themselves if they are being treated unfairly and also have the right to be happy in their employment.

There are also times when a parent may not feel confident approaching the school their child attends if something is wrong. They may think their child will then be treated differently by the staff and won't say anything. There is always a way where you can approach someone to resolve an issue.

If you are being discriminated against or being treated unfairly, you must stand up for yourself, otherwise the unfair treatment will continue.

WE CAN, SO WE MUST!

We all have the right to be happy with what we are doing and we all should be happy with our lives and the choices we have made.

Advocates can also work with people regarding their goal setting. For example, if someone wants to move out of home but their family feel they are not ready, an advocate will come in and work out a system of smaller goals to achieve before embarking on the larger goal of moving out of home. The advocate would assist the person in each smaller goal giving them the skills to move toward the larger goal.

When I have spoken about advocacy with people, a lot of them don't know what it is. They have never heard of advocacy.

As I mentioned previously, we all have the same rights as everyone else and we should all be able to stand up for those rights even if we need the assistance of someone else.

People with disabilities are not the only people that use advocacy services. Many people do not have the confidence or ability to stand up for their rights, which is why we all have access to advocacy services.

CHAPTER 13

OUR AMAZING BOY

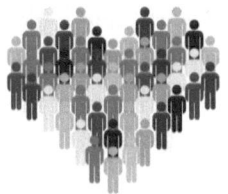

My son is super AWESOME
And I am the lucky one
Because I get to be his Mother.
HEALING HUGS

When Darcy was born, he was thrust into a world full of lots of people. Having two older brothers who were both in school, as well as playing football and basketball.

Right from the start he was exposed to people and people were exposed to him. All of our friends accepted him immediately for who he was, however, there were a few that only saw the Down Syndrome.

One of the comments that stands out to me was on the first day I took him to drop off the boys at school and we were surrounded by loads of women coming to see Darcy. (I have mentioned this story in *The Unexpected Journey*). Some were there as friends to meet Darcy and others were there to see what he looked like. I understood that because while I was pregnant, that was one of the things I thought about a lot.

Most people were gushing at how cute he was and giving me congratulations.

One lady however must have been asked if she knew me because I heard her response which was, 'Oh no, I've just come to see what he looks like'. I responded with, 'He looks like a baby'. She quickly retreated as she received stares from the others around Darcy and she was also embarrassed that I had actually heard what she said. Many were there to see what he looked like, but this lady was the only one that made the comment which was embarrassing and rude.

Darcy being exposed to such a social world was great to me because it showed people that he was just like any other baby. He was a little person who had joined our family.

Even though there were extra appointments for him and extra time with learning, at the end of the day, he was Darcy. A little boy who we had the same dreams and aspirations for as his older brothers.

Because he was in front of all these people and organisations, such as the school, Auskick, the basketball stadium, it was clear to me that if he wanted to, he should be able to have a go and try the same things his brothers did.

As he grew, and the more we did with him, I could see how with a little conversation and advocacy, people were willing to assist him and let him have a go. We did still come across some negativity, but when he shone, he did so very brightly.

I spoke a lot in my book *The Unexpected Journey* about the things Darcy participates in. All of these things, even the all-abilities programs, have been extremely inclusive experiences for him.

With the dual schooling, he got to learn on a different level to his special school such as being involved in a much larger class. He also got to do the same things his brothers did through his primary years. This school was amazingly supportive (with only a few hiccups and negative experiences), and Darcy did everything. He participated in all the specialty days, dress up days, excursions, incursions and camps. He attended all four camps, from Grade 3 to Grade 6. He also participated in the Year 6 Production *Olivia* and we could see how proud all of his friends were that he was part of that. Even though he only attended one day a week, the school made sure he could practise and he was included just like all the other children in their final year of primary school.

I did have to advocate heavily on his behalf when the Grade 3 camp was approaching. As mentioned earlier, there were many teachers at the school that thought he should not attend because he has Down Syndrome and they were worried about his ability. Every question asked by the school was answered clearly by me and the end result was the best outcome of him going to the camp.

When he returned from each camp, the teachers would come to me and say how wonderful he went and that he had participated in every single activity. In participating in the specialty days and camps, he was able to show many other people outside the school community how able he actually was.

I believe, for Darcy, being involved in mainstream schooling also definitely assisted with his gross and fine motor skills development as well as his speech. I am so happy we made the decision and had the support to send him there. He thoroughly enjoyed the seven years he was there and has also made some lifelong friends from the experience.

Darcy participates in dance with BAM Arts Inc, an all-abilities group that does dance, singing, arts, drama and provides many, many more wonderful opportunities for kids from the age of three. The age range in the group is from 3 to 60 plus and every one of the students at BAM thoroughly enjoys their time there.

BAM have a wonderful concert every year, attend community events, weekly challenges (which were a new thing during COVID-19), and many more fun inclusive things.

Being able to participate in community events is wonderful because so many different types of people have a chance to come and watch our amazing stars. They can see that at the end of the day they are expressive and like to show that they are able, and they enjoy the same things as everyone else. It shows the wider community they are people like everyone else.

Darcy is very sporty and participated in our local Auskick clinic for five years where the assistance required for him was no trouble at all from anyone. He was treated like every other child at the clinic (our local clinic is always in excess of 200 participants).

His time at Auskick also allowed him the opportunity to play football on the MCG and Marvel Stadium on several occasions. Again, nothing was too hard to accommodate his needs to be able to participate with the other children.

He plays basketball with the Westernport club in Special Olympics. He has participated in several regional and state events and was to represent Victoria in the Junior Nationals, but unfortunately due to COVID-19, the event has been cancelled. He would have participated in basketball and athletics at the Nationals where again, all the athletes would have been able to showcase their abilities. There will be more opportunities for him to represent his state in future years with Special Olympics.

Another love of Darcy's is bowling, and boy has he excelled in that over the last few years. He has gone from using a roller to bowl the ball, to the classic Fred Flintstone run up and bowl. It's lovely to see him gain new skills and enjoy what he is doing so much. He is now in two bowling competitions as well as social bowling with his carer and friends.

We love to go to concerts and the theatre, and one of my favourite things about that is the way he enjoys the performances so much. He doesn't worry about what people think if he cheers and claps and even gets up to dance. He just thoroughly enjoys the performances and gets so involved in what he is watching. I love this about him.

One of our favourite summer activities to attend is with the Disabled Surfers Association on the Mornington Peninsula. They run an amazingly inclusive day of volunteers assisting people of all abilities to try surfing. There is nobody that cannot attend this event. They make everything possible for people to be able to experience the fun of the surf and Darcy thoroughly enjoys riding the waves. The people that dedicate their time to make sure this event can happen are truly special.

An amazing person we have recently met is Louise Larkin who heads the wonderful inclusive organisation Friend In Me. They run fully inclusive events for everyone to attend and their mission is to ensure 'no child is left behind'. We have been fortunate to attend a couple of these events as well as quite a few online parties while face-to-face events weren't possible due to COVID-19. I love what her group represents and am honoured to call her my friend and be involved in her group. We are looking forward to attending more and more activities with her and Friend In Me and helping to raise awareness with them.

We have also been very fortunate to become involved with Stephanie Rodden's Celebrate T21 group, with Darcy being an ambassador for 2020. We were involved in many activities during the year and Darcy has been included in the amazing book they produce showing the wonderful world of Down Syndrome and raising awareness to show the beautiful people we call our family and friends. Stephanie provides gift care packages for new families of children with a diagnosis of Down Syndrome, and we are honoured to be part of this group with Darcy representing them and *The Unexpected Journey* being part of the packages the families receive.

Making Chromosomes Count is another organisation raising awareness and showcasing to the world the fascinating kaleidoscope that is Down Syndrome and its community. Darcy has been fortunate to become an ambassador for this group for 2021 and has featured on the front cover of their newly produced magazine. It is such a pleasure, and we are so proud that Darcy is a face people will recognise and also see his abilities. There are many opportunities with MCC to show the world the capabilities of everyone through articles, videos and other forms of social media sharing. MCC is based in England, but thanks to social media, we have been able to become part of this group and raise awareness with them globally.

Recently, we have been very fortunate to meet our local Federal Member Peta Murphy, and through her, Darcy was invited to be part of our local basketball team, The Frankston Blues training session.

Darcy was treated like any other young boy coming to watch his idols train. They have embraced him as one of their friends and attending training nights is now a regular occurrence. Wayne Holdsworth, the CEO of The Frankston Blues has also been wonderful and is creating employment opportunities for people living with a disability. The space at Frankston Blues is so inviting, inclusive and accepting. Darcy loves basketball and this has been a fantastic new event for him to go to every couple of weeks.

From these friendships with Peta Murphy, Wayne Holdsworth and The Frankston Blues, Darcy's dance group BAM are now performing at half-time of the home games and there are already things happening with the employment opportunities. There are many different roles someone could fulfill at this stadium and I am looking forward to seeing it all evolve.

One of the other things I love about my boy is the way he includes everyone around him. He doesn't judge or worry about what you look like. He accepts everyone for who they are and if he likes you, he includes you in everything he does.

There's no name calling or leaving people out because of what they can or can't do, or what they look like. It's wonderful and I think we can all learn a lesson from this.

I honestly wish more people were like Darcy and his friends. The world would be a much more harmonious place if they were.

My son, live your life to the fullest.
Spread your wings and fly high up in the air.
You can achieve much greater things
in your life because you are my son,
and I have put my Trust in you!
I love you son.
**PIXELSQUOTES.COM
(FOR MY 3 SONS)**

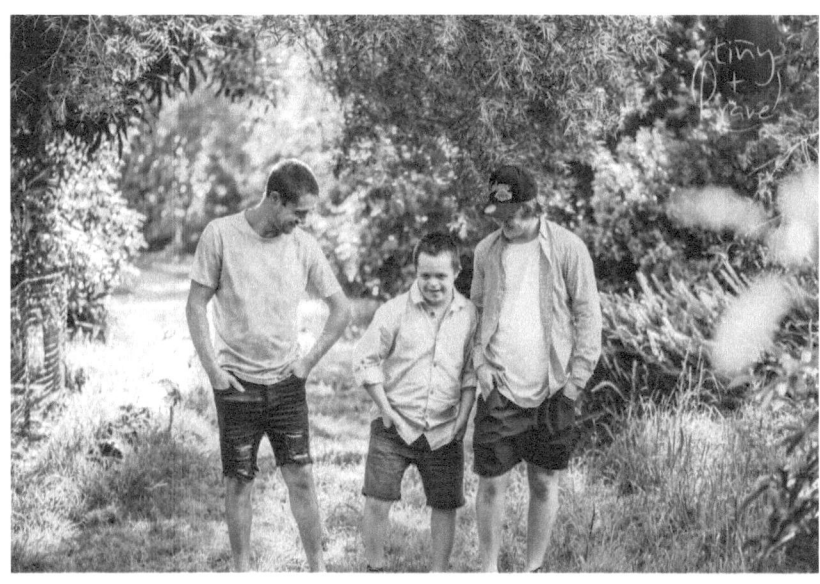

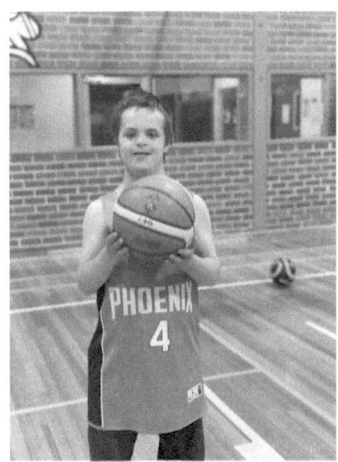
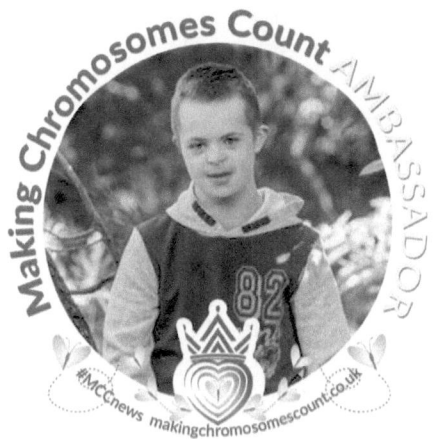
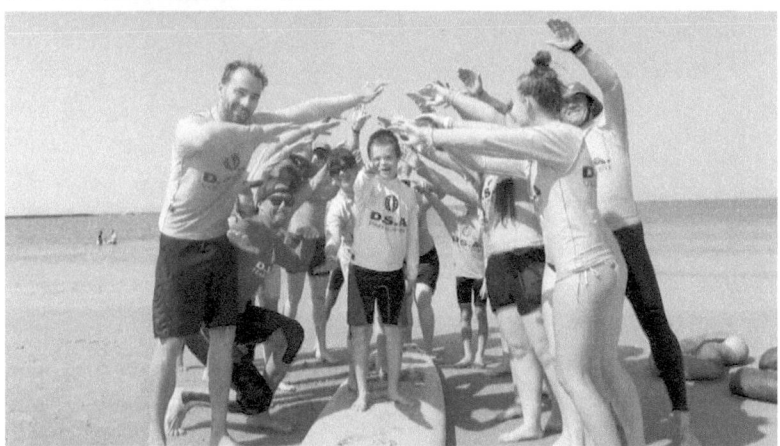
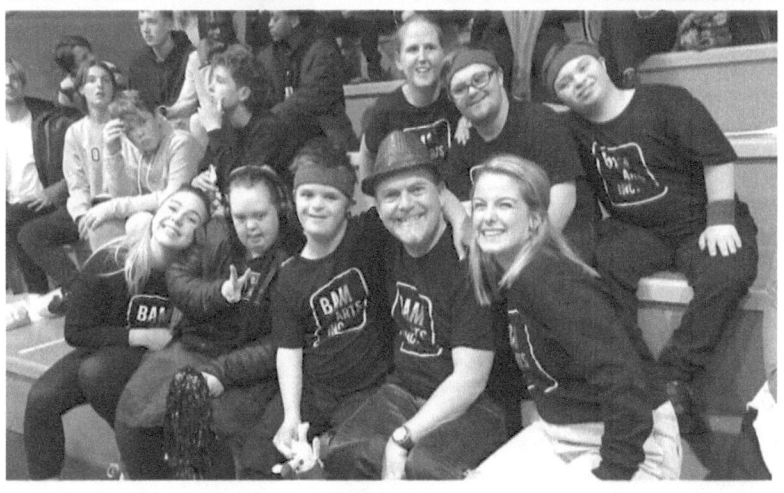

CHAPTER 14

FINAL THOUGHTS

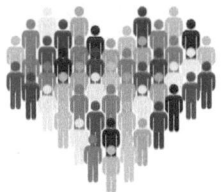

When you do learn these things, when you understand what inclusion is, then we can accomplish greater things together.

ALDIS HODGE

As a mum (and I mean to all my children, not just Darcy), it is so important for inclusion and acceptance to just be a part of everyday life.

It is important to me because I think when we do this, it gives people further confidence to put themselves forward for all sorts of things. It also gives their parents and carers the confidence to attend more events and put their children forward no matter what their ability is.

Support from others also helps this process.

> Peace requires everyone to be in the circle – wholeness, inclusion.
> **ISABELLE ALLENDE**

The support we got from the primary school for Darcy to attend part time was amazing. Even once he had started, the support from them gave me confidence to keep moving forward with the dual schooling. I remember saying to the principal I was happy he was doing this but knew that it would probably only last for 3–4 years and he wouldn't graduate from the school in Grade 6. I thought this because of the age gap that becomes bigger as the kids get older because of Darcy's delayed learning capabilities.

His response was, 'Why can't he graduate? We will make sure that he gets every opportunity to make that happen'.

WOW! That blew my mind and gave me a newfound confidence to keep going and keep pushing so that he got the same opportunities as his brothers, and also to teach him and others it's okay to be different, and that everybody has different abilities.

It is important for me because I have witnessed time and time again, that when we include and accept others, it makes everyone feel good about themselves. We see many more smiles from people when they feel like they should be there, when they feel like they can and when they feel like they are not being judged.

FINAL THOUGHTS

When you judge another, you do not define them. You define yourself.
AUTHOR UNKNOWN

It is important to remember to not just invite someone to the party … this is only part of inclusion. The rest of this, and to make someone feel like they really belong, is to also dance with them.

There is no point including someone in an activity (such as a party or a sport) if you are not going to interact with them as well.

When we go out, we all like to interact and be social with others. People with disabilities are no different. Actually, nobody is any different This is something we all like to do.

We want a culture that is inclusive of everyone and where everyone who joins feels they have opportunities to succeed and grow.
NELLIE BORRERO

FROM THE HEARTS AND MINDS OF MUMS

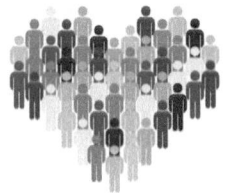

I approached some friends of mine and asked them if they would be willing to answer some questions to give people a better understanding of what inclusion means to them.

I asked six questions and had five friends take part in providing me with answers. Please take time to read their answers and see how certain things make them feel and what they would like others to know.

Tina Naughton – Mum to Amy (diagnosis – Down Syndrome)

1. What does inclusion mean to you?

Inclusion to me means that you are accepted and embraced for the person you are.

2. How confident are you putting your child forward for activities?

To be honest, I am more than happy to put Amy forward for an activity, when someone else is going to take her; because I know that she will behave for other's when I am not around.

If I was to put her forward for an activity where I had to be the one engaging her that would be a whole different story. It would be very much dependant on my state of mind at the time, and whether I had the 'mental' energy to keep her engaged in that activity.

3. How confident are you taking your child out shopping?

I have no problem taking Amy out shopping; we have been going to the same shopping centre since the day she was born. The staff have come to know her quite well and often say 'hi' to her and ask her how she's going. She's very sociable most of the time and quite often will initiate conversations with people. If they don't understand what she is saying or asking, I will explain what she is enquiring about and the same happens in reverse. If a person asks Amy a question, I will try to explain to Amy what they are asking and try to answer their question at the same time.

As far as her behaviour whilst shopping, she pretty much does what every other kid does and wants things that she's not allowed to have, and more often than not, I will find things in the trolley whilst at the register that she has put in there when I haven't been looking.

4. What are the things that may stop you from taking your child to participate in activities?

Amy's behaviours at times can be very stressful and challenging to say the least. She is blindingly stubborn, so much so, there are times when I just say 'no' to invites. I choose the easy 'stay at home' option rather than go out, and have to fight to keep her interested in what we are doing. It's not that we are trying to make her do anything dangerous, or something we wouldn't ordinarily do; just a nice walk at the beach or visit a friend for a cuppa and a chat, sit down and have a picnic. No, if she doesn't want to do it, she makes such a fuss, people nearby, would think we are trying to hurt her. Socialising with like-minded friends and their kids around certainly does help quell the situation sometimes, but ultimately, we do get to a point of 'enough is enough!' We pick up our gear and go home and she returns to the happy, smiling Amy again.

There was a time I tried to get her involved in a dance class; because I thought she would enjoy the company of her friends as well as the movement to music. She sat on the floor and refused to move, and when I tried to get her up, she promptly laid herself on the floor and made it impossible to get her to her feet. It wasn't until I said we were going home, that she got herself off the floor and made her way outside.

I know I shouldn't worry about what other people think, but I do. It's human nature. And unfortunately, people do make the assumption that the bad behaviour is because of their disability, and often say, 'Oh … she doesn't understand what she's doing'. Believe me that makes it all the more frustrating, because Amy is very much aware of how she should, or shouldn't behave.

5. How does it make you feel when your child is being excluded?

I have never been able to deal with her being excluded.

Outwardly I act confidently, and deal with it the best way I can at the time; internally it absolutely breaks my heart.

One occasion that always comes to my mind, and to this very day, still upsets me when I think about it; a youngster thought it funny to lock her in a cubby house, then run off and leave her there, and then laugh at her efforts when she's calling for help and trying to get out. Fortunately, we weren't too far away and heard her calling and saw this youngster laughing at her.

When questioned if they had locked her in there and who their parents were, they shrugged their shoulders as if they had done nothing wrong, grinned and ran off like it was some sort of a joke. It happened at a friend's birthday party, so there were lots of kids, and parents around, completely unaware of what had taken place; then a few weeks later, at a similar sort of gathering, I walked in on a conversation where a group of children were having a laugh at Amy's expense, and that was it. I'd had enough, couldn't cope with it; as a consequence, over a period of time, I quietly, and without any explanation, distanced myself from the group. I couldn't find a way past trying to explain why I had distanced myself. I'm certain they would have empathised; the hurt, however, was very real for us, and I kept knocking back invitations with all sorts of excuses until the invitations stopped.

6. What would you like to say to the wider public to raise awareness about inclusion?

Please understand, they are people first; their disability is only part of them. They have the same emotions, worries and concerns like the rest of us.

Please ask questions before making assumptions about what they can or cannot do. It may come as a surprise to many people, if they took the time to find out more about members of our community who live with a disability, that they are quite 'able' to do many things. It may take some of them a little longer to learn a skill. They, like everyone have the capability to learn.

Tanya Thomas – Mum to Teagan & Seth (diagnosis – autism)

1. What does inclusion mean to you?

Inclusion to me means every person regardless of disabilities, or any differences should be included in opportunities and everyday things to feel part of their community and their world. As parents and carers we shouldn't have to advocate so much for inclusion.

2. How confident are you putting your child forward for activities?

I am very confident now but this wasn't always the case.

3. How confident are you taking your child out shopping?

Still not very confident, more due to my child escaping to a dangerous car park or road, though not really about how other people may comment or stare.

4. What are the things that may stop you from taking your child to participate in activities?

Parks that are not correctly fenced with barriers to roads or waterways, or businesses that are not disability inclusive.

5. How does it make you feel when your child is being excluded?

Sad, because no-one should ever be made to feel this way.

6. What would you say to the wider public to raise awareness about inclusion?

Inclusion should not be something that needs to be fought for, we should not need to be reminding the community as often as we do. There is plenty of disability awareness nowadays – we need to work on disability acceptance and inclusion.

Tracey O'Brien – Mum to Lilly (diagnosis Down Syndrome/Autism)

1. What does inclusion mean to you?

Being accepted for who you are and not feeling left out or judged.

2. How confident are you putting your child forward for activities?

I am not confident whatsoever because of my own anxiety and my daughter's and the fear of being judged.

3. How confident are you taking your child out shopping?

Not confident whatsoever and actually refuse to take her at the fear of being stared at, judged, ridiculed and hearing negative comments.

4. What are the things that may stop you from taking your child to participate in activities?

Worrying about what others think. Anxiety. Her challenging behaviours and anxiety.

5. How does it make you feel when your child is being excluded?

It makes me feel gutted and a failure as a mum. It makes me upset for her feelings. I don't like to see anyone being excluded because I think everyone deserves a chance.

6. What would you like to say to the wider public to raise awareness about inclusion?

People that live with disabilities are people first; their disability is only part of them. See the person, not the disability.

Always know that parents are open to people asking questions rather than making assumptions or staring and pointing. We would much rather this, believe me.

It hurts us as parents to think that our children aren't being regarded as equal to everyone else. They have the same rights as all of us and should be treated this way.

Anonymous

1. What does inclusion mean to you?

To me, inclusion means giving people a chance. Inviting them to take part and then working with them to allow them to be involved. If inviting someone to a party, you need to also dance with them to make them feel a part of the party, not just have them there.

2. How confident are you putting your child forward for activities?

I am much more confident now my child is older and in their teens. There are still times when I am anxious to put them forward for activities due to the fear of them being judged, jeered at and pointed at. It really depends on where we are going and who we are with.

3. How confident are you taking your child out shopping?

My child loves to come shopping, however, I avoid it where I can. I find that I cannot handle people staring at them. My child looks different to others and is quite noisy while out.

I find people moving aside, staring and pointing and I don't like it. I would rather do the shopping by myself to avoid this.

When I get home my child always helps me pack things away and loves to look at everything I brought home.

4. What are the things that may stop you from taking your child to participate in activities?

The main thing here is worrying that my child will feel as though they shouldn't be there because of staring, pointing and others not including them.

Feeling alone while trying to participate in an activity isn't fun.

5. How does it make you feel when your child is being excluded?

I actually feel a little sorry for the people making them feel excluded. My child is a fun loving, beautifully natured person and they are missing out on all the wonderful traits they have.

My child loves to be social and when they are excluded, I feel very sad and sometimes angry. I don't understand it at all.

My heart breaks for my child because they are at the age now where they fully understand being excluded. I don't like the way it makes them feel.

6. What would you like to say to the wider public to raise awareness about inclusion?

I would like to say to the wider public that everyone is different. We live in a very diverse world and we should embrace everyone for their differences.

We are all different, but we do all have the same wants and needs.

Please look at the person and not the disability. Understand that we all have the same feelings.

Tanya Todd – Mum to Evan (diagnosis ASD/intellectual disability/ADHD/Dyspraxia

1. What does inclusion mean to you?

When I think of inclusion, I don't necessarily think of being included in an activity or task specifically, although that is definitely part of it.

I think of acceptance and a feeling of belonging. Being treated with the same respect and empathy as everybody else.

I think of being able to feel at ease and comfortable in any situation or at any place. An understanding that we all have differences and that is okay. Each of us need to treat everyone with kindness.

Inclusion is being able to adapt situations, activities and experiences so that everyone feels that they belong.

2. How confident are you putting your child forward for activities?

I am pretty confident putting my son forward for activities, but sometimes it's hard not knowing how he will respond. He can become very stubborn and defiant and this leads to a negative aversion to the activity.

He often chooses not to try and this makes me sad. It can also cause others to look and stare which also makes both of us feel uncomfortable.

3. How confident are you taking your child out shopping?

My son loves shopping, but once he's done, he's done. He is a very helpful shopper, and sometimes we end up with a few extras in our trolley … he he!

If it's not food shopping, he is less tolerant unless it is for him. I need to discuss exactly what we need to buy and which shops we will go to for it to be successful. I often leave Evan's part of the shopping trip until the end to stretch him out as long as I can.

When he was younger, it was not so successful. He would bolt or drop and starfish. It was stressful and caused me great anxiety.

I had a planned speech in my head ready to say to people if we experienced any stares or comments. My speech to others was – 'You don't know him and you don't know me. We don't affect your life, so please keep your judgement to yourself and keep living it!'

But, I never had the courage to say it. I would tell myself if I was having anxiety about going out, if I hide my child from the world, then I will hide the world from my child. And that's not what I wanted to do.

I am glad I found the courage to do things that were out of my comfort zone because he has learned so much and welcomes so many fun adventures.

4. What are the things that may stop you from taking your child to participate in activities?

When he was younger, I would worry about his stubbornness and the way he reacted when he didn't want to do something. He would run off from me or drop to the ground.

This caused unwanted looks, pointing and comments from others which made me feel very anxious.

As he has become older and more understanding of the activities we are doing, it is definitely less stressful. I will talk to him about what we are going to do and try and make him aware of what it is before we get there. I find this helps with his anxiety and makes the trip more successful.

5. How does it make you feel when your child is being excluded?

When I can see that my child is being excluded, it makes me feel sad, angry and anxious. It breaks my heart.

My son is quite intuitive, and he knows when people are not being kind. He gets quite upset, cries and runs off to hide.

It takes a long time to help him feel better because he then becomes embarrassed at his reaction. When he is embarrassed, he won't let anyone console him. It's just heartbreaking.

6. What would you like to say to the wider public to raise awareness about inclusion?

Evan participated in a program with his school where they included two specialist classrooms in a mainstream school. It was a program to build relationships, experiences and inclusion.

Once when we were out at our local Pet's Day Out, we saw one of the girls from the mainstream part of the school with her mother.

She knew my son from the school, and I heard her say to her mum, 'That boy goes to my school – he's weird'.

I will never forget how sad and infuriated this made me feel.

I wanted to say to the mother, 'Aren't you going to say something to her? Aren't you going to explain that this is not okay?'

My son heard her, I heard her, and her mother heard her. This was a wasted opportunity to educate her child and tell her how unkind her words were. By saying nothing at all, she was teaching her child that it's okay to say such things and be unkind.

We need to teach our children to accept people for who they are and if they can't do that, just leave them alone. No need for comments like this.

AHA MOMENTS AND TAKEAWAYS

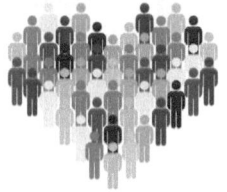

I hope, after reading *The Magic of Inclusion*, you have gained an insight into what some families deal with daily. And I hope you can encourage others to be kind.

Remember, it is not only people who live with a disability that experience exclusion, it happens to many people every day. I have written about acceptance and inclusion from my experiences with my son Darcy and also from my friends who have shared stories with me.

Next time you see someone who lives with a disability out and about, please …

- Smile
- Say hello
- If they look like they need some help, offer them a hand
- If it is a mum who looks as though she is struggling, offer her some help and support
- Remember everyone has the same dreams and aspirations
- Include the person you see being left out
- BE KIND
- See the 'person' first, not their disability

If you are a parent who struggles to take their children out because of how others make you feel, please …

- Don't stay at home
- Take your child out and enjoy activities
- Take someone with you
- Use your support worker to go with you
- Try and smile at the people staring
- Say hello to others
- Be proud of 'you' and your child

And please don't forget to …

GIVE PEOPLE A CHANCE AND WATCH THEM SHINE

AFTERWORD

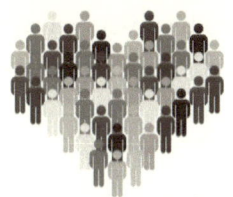

My aim in writing this book, is to show people how important inclusion and acceptance is in our society. With people living with a disability and also with everyone. Many people experience exclusion, not only people living with a disability.

I want people to stop and think before they do something toward someone else and I want them to put themselves in their shoes to try and get an understanding of what it may feel like to be treated differently.

I want people to put the shoe on the other foot and think about how they would feel if they, or someone they love like their child, were being made to feel as though they shouldn't be where they are enjoying things like everyone else.

I also want parents to gain confidence to take their children out and about in society and make wonderful memories with them. I don't want people to worry about where they can or cannot take their child because of what others may say to them.

It took me a long time to ignore stares and snide remarks about my son. Believe me, it has taken a lot of strength and there are still occasions where I do let my guard down and comment to people how rude they are being.

But when I allow myself to be upset by others, it takes away precious enjoyable time with my son.

It is hard sometimes, but I now choose to ignore comments or try and make a positive comment back to them and when I feel people staring at my son, I smile at them or say hello. The end result of me doing this, is that we get to continue on our way in a positive mindset and enjoy the day ahead.

We all have different experiences and stories to share, but at the end of the day, we just want our children to enjoy life and not worry about the negativity of others. Please be the person that steps up and stops exclusion from happening.

I hope that by writing this book, people will look at the person first, not their disability. People live with a disability … it is part of them. It is NOT who they are.

Why do I want to raise awareness on inclusion and acceptance?

His name is Darcy and he is my son.

AFTERWORD

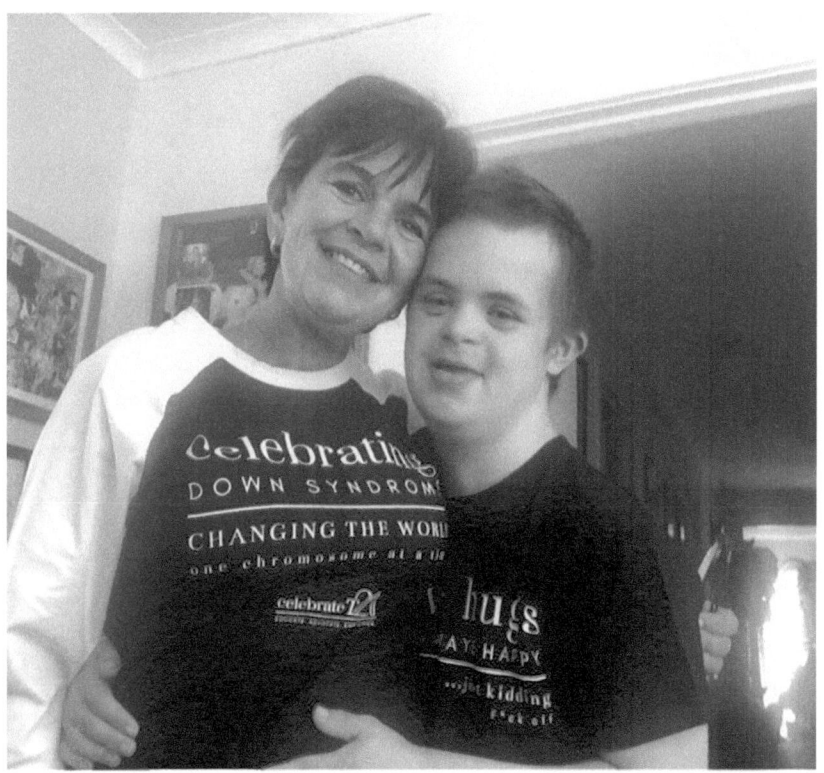

Please understand I have a disability, not a disease. You can't catch it. I may walk, talk, and move differently than you do, but on the inside I am not so different.
CHARISSE, LIVING WITH CEREBRAL PALSY

ABOUT THE AUTHOR

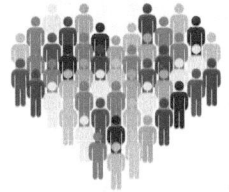

Julie Fisher is wife to Mick, Mum to Caleb, Blake and Darcy, Stepmum to Bree and she is also a carer for her son Darcy.

After completing her dream of writing her first book *The Unexpected Journey: Embracing the Beauty of Disability*, a burning passion was ignited to do more within the Down Syndrome community and also for others living with a disability.

Since completing her first book, Julie has worked together with other disability groups such as Down Syndrome Australia and Down Syndrome Victoria, and has been part of the Truly Incredible Care Campaign in 2020 with Carers Victoria.

She has written many articles which have been published on media platforms online. She has spoken about her journey with her son Darcy in the hope to raise awareness in the wider community.

Julie saw a need to raise awareness around inclusion and acceptance for people with disabilities (and for many others), and decided it was time to publish her second book, to show people that everyone should have a chance to be included and accepted and live life just like everybody else.

Her mentors and employers Stuart and Natasa Denman and work colleague Vivienne Mason have helped her to keep pursuing her dreams of working with families and raising much needed awareness, and have been the driving force behind her completing her books.

She enjoys speaking about her journey and spreading the message of awareness for people living with a disability and can be contacted at her website www.juliefisher.com.au

Julie's hope is for everyone to be treated fairly and the same, and to enjoy life's adventures.

> Writing a book is not about the book,
> it's about the person you become at the other end.
> **NATASA DENMAN**
> **ULTIMATE 48 HOUR AUTHOR**

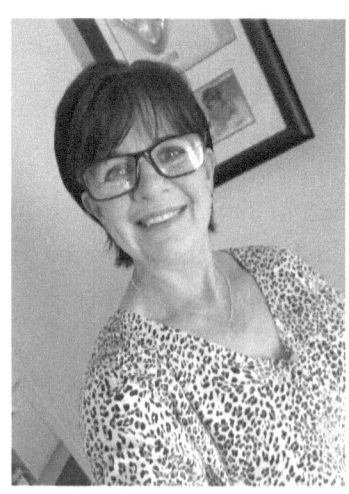

ACKNOWLEDGEMENTS

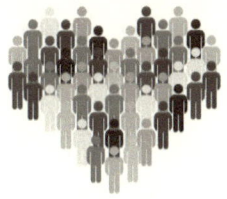

I would like thank and acknowledge the following people for their contributions to this book:

Members of the group Dance With Down Syndrome for contributing to the chapter that talks about language and what people have said to them about their children.

My friends:

Tina Naughton

Tanya Thomas

Tracey O'Brien

Tanya Todd

For their contribution to the questions asked about inclusion.

Many of my friends have experienced exclusion with their children and I think it's important to hear from them. They are our children, we love them and want to protect them from being treated in this way. It is important for this to stop.

Thank you all from the bottom of my heart for contributing to this book to give people a better understanding of living with a disability and the importance of inclusion and acceptance.

To Louise Larkin, founder of Friend In Me – thank you so much for contributing to this book with the foreword you wrote. You and I both have the same passion and drive to raise awareness about inclusion and acceptance. We met two years ago, and I love doing things with you and supporting your wonderful organisation.

OFFERS

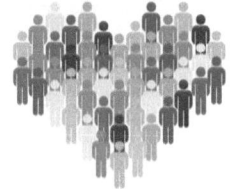

ARE YOU INCLUSIVE ENOUGH?

Would you like a consultation for resources and strategies to become more inclusive?

Take the survey here –

Businesses – https://tinyurl.com/1business-survey

Take the survey here –

Schools – https://tinyurl.com/1school-survey

FOR MUMS & DADS
Download your free sheet here with ideas and strategies for your children

https://tinyurl.com/mumsanddadspdf

OFFERS

FOR BUSINESSES

Download your free tips sheet for inclusion tips to make your business accepting, inclusive and accessible.

https://tinyurl.com/business-tipsheet

FOR SCHOOLS

Download your free tips sheet for strategies on inclusion in the school.

https://tinyurl.com/schooltipsheet

THE MAGIC OF INCLUSION

Follow Julie at The Unexpected Journey on Facebook

by scanning the QR Code

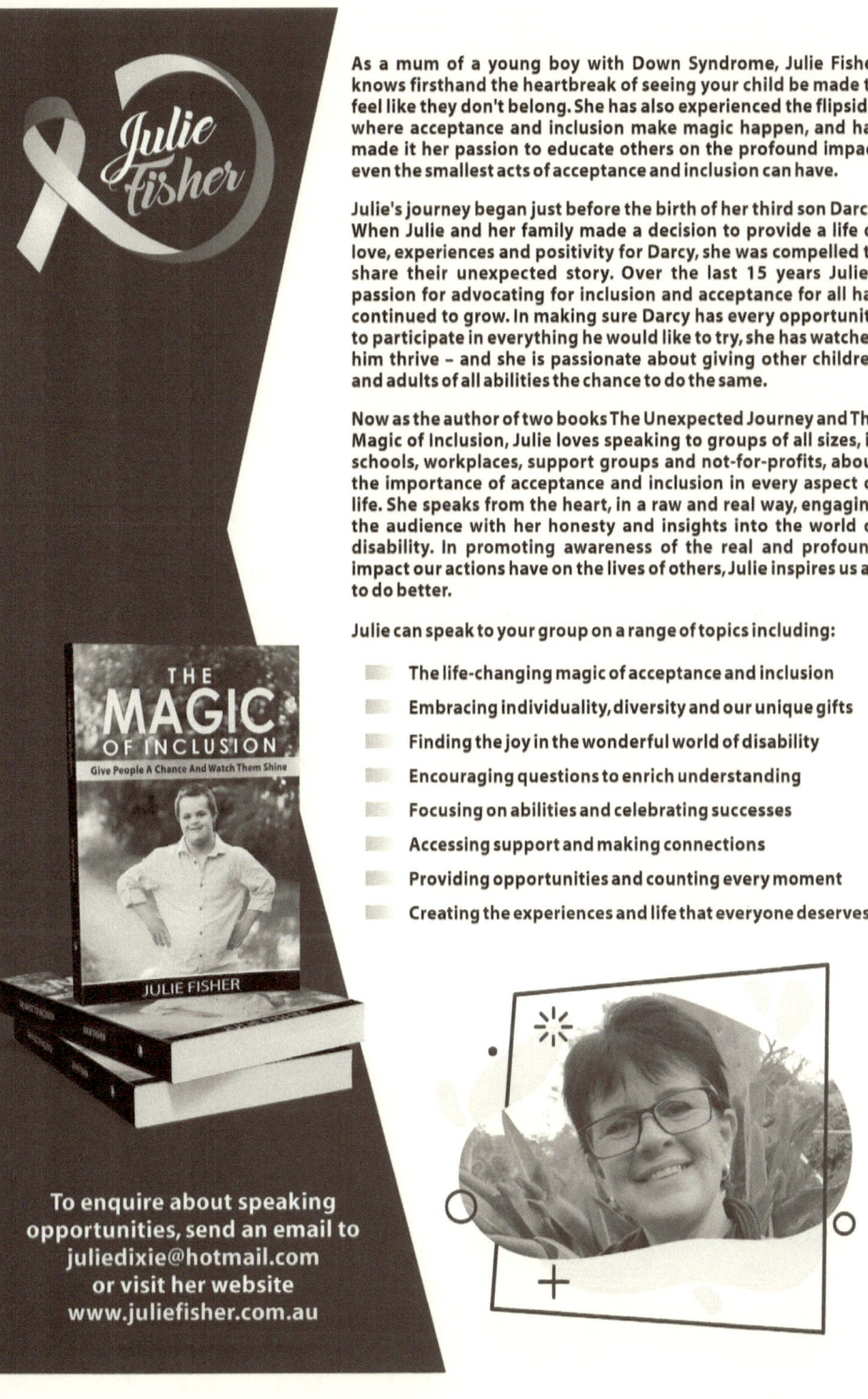

As a mum of a young boy with Down Syndrome, Julie Fisher knows firsthand the heartbreak of seeing your child be made to feel like they don't belong. She has also experienced the flipside, where acceptance and inclusion make magic happen, and has made it her passion to educate others on the profound impact even the smallest acts of acceptance and inclusion can have.

Julie's journey began just before the birth of her third son Darcy. When Julie and her family made a decision to provide a life of love, experiences and positivity for Darcy, she was compelled to share their unexpected story. Over the last 15 years Julie's passion for advocating for inclusion and acceptance for all has continued to grow. In making sure Darcy has every opportunity to participate in everything he would like to try, she has watched him thrive – and she is passionate about giving other children and adults of all abilities the chance to do the same.

Now as the author of two books The Unexpected Journey and The Magic of Inclusion, Julie loves speaking to groups of all sizes, in schools, workplaces, support groups and not-for-profits, about the importance of acceptance and inclusion in every aspect of life. She speaks from the heart, in a raw and real way, engaging the audience with her honesty and insights into the world of disability. In promoting awareness of the real and profound impact our actions have on the lives of others, Julie inspires us all to do better.

Julie can speak to your group on a range of topics including:

- The life-changing magic of acceptance and inclusion
- Embracing individuality, diversity and our unique gifts
- Finding the joy in the wonderful world of disability
- Encouraging questions to enrich understanding
- Focusing on abilities and celebrating successes
- Accessing support and making connections
- Providing opportunities and counting every moment
- Creating the experiences and life that everyone deserves

To enquire about speaking opportunities, send an email to juliedixie@hotmail.com or visit her website www.juliefisher.com.au

If you see someone falling behind, walk beside them.
If you see someone being ignored, find a way to include them.
Always remind people of their worth.
One small act could mean the world to them.

AUTHOR UNKNOWN

LINKS FOR SUPPORT SERVICES AND ORGANISATIONS THAT PROMOTE INCLUSION THAT WE HAVE USED AND ARE PART OF

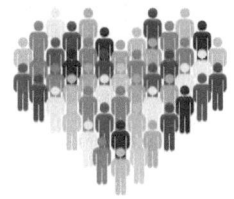

Carers Victoria - https://www.carersvictoria.org.au/

Friend In Me - https://www.friendinme.org.au/

Happiness First - https://www.happinessfirst.com.au/

Down Syndrome Victoria - https://www.downsyndrome.org.au/vic/

Down Syndrome Australia - https://www.downsyndrome.org.au/

Association for Children with a Disability - https://www.acd.org.au/

Children and Young People With Disability Australia - https://www.cyda.org.au/

Youth Disability Advocacy Service - https://www.yacvic.org.au/ydas/

Celebrate T21 - https://celebratet21.com/

Keeley's Cause - https://keeleyscause.org.au/

Making Chromosome Count – The DS Community News - http://www.makingchromosomescount.co.uk/

ABILITY
is what you're capable of doing

MOTIVATION
determines what you do

ATTITUDE
determines how well you do it

NOTES

THE MAGIC OF INCLUSION

NOTES

www.ingramcontent.com/pod-product-compliance
Lightning Source LLC
Chambersburg PA
CBHW021437080526
44588CB00009B/568